Introductory Guide to Cardiac CT Imaging

Introductory Guide to Cardiac CT Imaging

Ragavendra R. Baliga, MD, MBA, FRCP, FACC

Vice Chief & Assistant Division Director
Division of Cardiovascular Medicine
Professor of Internal Medicine
The Ohio State University
Columbus, Ohio

Wolters Kluwer | Lippincott Williams & Wilkins
Health

Philadelphia · Baltimore · New York · London
Buenos Aires · Hong Kong · Sydney · Tokyo

Acquisitions Editor: Frances R. DeStefano
Product Manager: Leanne McMillan
Production Manager: Alicia Jackson
Senior Manufacturing Manager: Benjamin Rivera
Marketing Manager: Kimberly Schonberger
Design Coordinator: Teresa Mallon
Production Service: Aptara, Inc.

Printed in China

Library of Congress Cataloging-in-Publication Data

Introductory guide to cardiac CT imaging / [edited by] Ragavendra R. Baliga.
    p. ; cm.
Includes bibliographical references.
ISBN 978-1-58255-938-4
1. Heart—Tomography. I. Baliga, R. R.
[DNLM: 1. Coronary Artery Disease—radiography. 2. Tomography, X-Ray Computed—
methods. 3. Coronary Angiography—methods. WG 141.5.T6 I616 2010]
RC683.5.T66I58 2010
616.1′20757—dc22

                                                                        2009015265

To purchase additional copies of this book, call our customer service department at
(800) 638-3030 or fax orders to (301) 223-2320. International customers should
call (301) 223-2300.

Visit Lippincott Williams & Wilkins on the Internet: at LWW.com. Lippincott Williams &
Wilkins customer service representatives are available from 8:30 am to 6 pm, EST.

This book is dedicated to Jayashree, Anoop, and Neena.

CONTRIBUTORS

Alex J. Auseon, DO
Assistant Professor of Clinical Medicine
Division of Cardiovascular Medicine
The Ohio State University Medical Center
Columbus, Ohio

Ragavendra R. Baliga, MD, MBA, FACC, FRCP
Vice Chief & Assistant Division Director
Division of Cardiovascular Medicine
Professor of Internal Medicine
The Ohio State University
Columbus, Ohio

Quinn Capers IV, MD, FACC, FSCAI
Associate Dean of Medicine
Director, Peripheral Vascular Interventions
Division of Cardiovascular Medicine
The Ohio State University Medical Center
Columbus, Ohio

Ernest L. Mazzaferri, Jr., MD
Assistant Professor of Cardiovascular Medicine
The Ohio State University
Ross Heart Hospital
Columbus, Ohio

Laxmi S. Mehta, MD

Assistant Professor of Clinical Medicine

Department of Internal Medicine, Division of Cardiovascular Medicine

The Ohio State University

Director, Women's Cardiovascular Health Clinic

Department of Internal Medicine, Division of Cardiovascular Medicine

The Ohio State University Medical Center

Columbus, Ohio

Subha V. Raman, MD, MSEE, FACC

Associate Professor of Internal Medicine

The Ohio State University

Medical Director, Cardiac CT/MR

Ohio State University Health System

Columbus, Ohio

Chittoor B. Sai Sudhakar, MBBS, FRCS, FACS

Assistant Professor of Surgery

Division of Cardiothoracic Surgery

The Ohio State University Medical Center

Attending Surgeon, Cardiothoracic Surgery

Richard M. Ross Heart Hospital and The Ohio State University Medical Center

Columbus, Ohio

Raul Weiss, MD FACC, FAHA, FHRS, CCDS
Associate Professor of Clinical Medicine and Cardiovascular
  Medicine
Director, Electrophysiology Fellowship Program
Cardiovascular Division
The Ohio State University
Ross Heart Hospital
Columbus, Ohio

PREFACE

Cardiac CT has recently emerged as an important diagnostic tool in the armamentarium of a practicing physician. With the development of ultrafast CT scanners and innovative techniques to minimize radiation exposure (to <5 mSv of radiation), this diagnostic modality should gain widespread acceptance.

This book serves to provide essential knowledge to the practicing physician who desires a rapid overview of this modality. The content of this book is unique in that the contributors are not only cardiologists who interpret and perform cardiac CT procedures but also those who regularly utilize this technique in their clinical practice. This unique perspective should provide a more comprehensive approach to those who are planning to increasingly utilize cardiac CT in their practice or planning to setup a cardiac CT facility in their office.

This book should be particularly useful to cardiologists, primary care physicians, internists, physician extenders, residents, medical students, nurses, and cardiovascular technicians who want a quick primer on this rapidly emerging modality.

Ragavendra R. Baliga, MD, MBA, FACC, FRCP (Edin), FRS MED
Vice-Chief, Division of Cardiovascular Medicine
Professor of Internal Medicine
The Ohio State University Medical Center

ACKNOWLEDGMENTS

I thank Jakki Vaughn and Teri Henderson, for helping me with my day-to-day logistics.

I thank Frances DeStefano from LWW for inviting me to do this book and Leanne McMillan for ensuring that this project comes to fruition. Finally, I thank Samir Roy for the excellent project management of this book.

CONTENTS

Introductory Guide to Cardiac CT Imaging

Indications

Ragavendra R. Baliga

INDICATIONS FOR CORONARY COMPUTED TOMOGRAPHY ANGIOGRAPHY

To rule out coronary stenosis in patients with low-to-intermediate risk of having coronary artery disease (CAD).

To rule out coronary stenosis in patients with inconsistent cardiac symptoms or inconsistent ischemia test results.

To evaluate bypass graft patency.

To evaluate bypass grafts not visualized by conventional angiography.

To evaluate coronary anomalies.

To evaluate coronary anatomy in new-onset heart failure.

To map coronary arteries and assess internal mammary arteries prior to re-do coronary artery bypass grafting.

CORONARY COMPUTED TOMOGRAPHY ANGIOGRAPHY IS *NOT* INDICATED IN THESE CONDITIONS CURRENTLY

To determine coronary stenosis in patients with high pretest probability of CAD.

To evaluate patients with unstable or acute coronary syndrome.

To evaluate coronary stent patency.

To evaluate myocardial viability and perfusion.

To screen healthy, asymptomatic individuals for exclusion of CAD.

CARDIAC COMPUTED TOMOGRAPHY

To evaluate cardiac mass when the images are technically limited with echocardiography, transesophageal echocardiogram, or magnetic resonance imaging.

To evaluate pulmonary vein anatomy for radiofrequency ablation of atrial fibrillation.

To map coronary veins for placement of biventricular pacemakers.

To evaluate suspected aortic aneurysm or aortic dissection.

To evaluate pericardial conditions (constrictive pericarditis, pericardial mass, complications of cardiac surgery) when the images are technically limited with echocardiography, transesophageal echocardiogram, or magnetic resonance imaging.

CHAPTER 2

Calcium Scoring: A Primer

Laxmi S. Mehta

INTRODUCTORY CONCEPTS

Coronary artery disease (CAD) is the leading cause of mortality in developed nations, however there are effective interventions that treat and retard CAD progression. Unfortunately, a large number of people are asymptomatic prior to presenting with an acute myocardial infarction or sudden cardiac death and therefore they lack access to the necessary preventative treatment. Early identification of subclinical atherosclerosis is imperative for risk stratification and early intervention to reduce cardiac events. Many risk factors for CAD have been identified, yet they are frequently interdependent of each other; for example, the Framingham Risk Score calculates the 10-year risk of CAD based on age, sex, smoking status, total cholesterol, HDL, and diabetes and hypertension history. Presence of coronary artery calcium on computed tomography (CT) images is independently associated with atherosclerotic plaque. Calcium scoring is a simple, reproducible test that can be used to identify atherosclerotic plaque even at an early stage, thereby warranting early implementation of treatment.

Any degree of calcium within the coronary tree implies atherosclerosis, as it is the only known process to cause deposition of calcium within the arterial wall (intima), occurring many years prior to the development of hemodynamically significant obstruction and symptoms. Specialized cells associated with bone remodeling, which are similar to bone-forming osteoblast cells, actively deposit calcium within the arterial wall. Arterial calcification is not due to a degenerative process (i.e., not caused by aging), yet it is associated with aging. Younger patients frequently lack calcium deposition, while elderly patients more likely than not have some degree of arterial calcification.

Coronary calcium scoring is a quantitative measure of the extent of atherosclerotic plaque burden, yet an important concept to remember is that it does not provide information on the degree of arterial luminal narrowing. Calcium scoring provides anatomical data that indicate the presence or absence of calcium within the coronary artery tree, whereas a stress test offers physiologic data that identify significant obstruction to coronary artery blood flow. Calcification in the coronary arteries can help detect atherosclerosis early in the process, even before the plaque becomes obstructive; therefore, CAD is identified on a CT scan much earlier than it would be on a stress test. Calcium is present within the intima of both obstructive and nonobstructive lesions; hence coronary calcification is specific for atheromatous plaque (Fig. 2-1) but is not specific for an obstructive lesion. In addition, progression of atherosclerosis can be monitored by tracking the change in calcium score over time in cohorts of patients who have or have not received interventions such as lipid therapy or lifestyle modification.

METHODOLOGY

CT has rapidly undergone changes over the last decade or more. Noncontrast CT is a quick imaging modality that uses

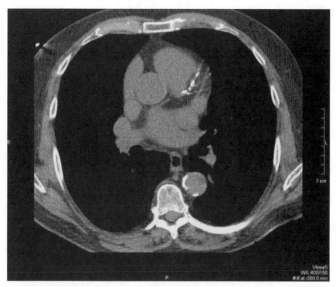

FIGURE 2-1. Sixteen-slice multidetector CT (MDCT) image showing calcium deposits in the left main, left anterior descending, diagonal, and proximal circumflex coronary arteries. (Reproduced from Higgins CB, de Roos A. MRI and CT of the Cardiovascular System, 2nd Ed. Philadelphia: Lippincott Williams & Wilkins 2006.)

low radiation dose and no contrast to detect coronary calcium within 10–15 minutes. Electron-beam computed tomography (EBCT) scanners use ultrafast scan acquisition times of 100 ms in synchrony with the heart cycle. The multisource detector is stationary while the electron beam sweeps across the tungsten rings. Thirty to 40 serial 3-mm-thick slice tomographic sections of the heart are acquired. The scan is obtained in one to two breath-holding sequences and is triggered with prospective gating. Multidetector computed tomography (MDCT) scanners uses multidetector rows to acquire multiple adjacent slices of the heart simultaneously. The x-ray photons are generated within an x-ray tube that houses a tungsten filament, which allows adjustment of the tube current (i.e., increase the number of photons for improved tissue penetration and diminished image noise in obese patients). The x-ray tube and opposing detectors rotate within the gantry. Images are acquired with either prospective or retrospective gating. The effective radiation dose for EBCT scans is 0.7 to 1.0 mSv in men and 0.9 to 1.3 mSv in women, and for MDCT scans it is 1 to 1.5 mSv in men and 1.1 to 1.8 mSv in women.[1]

EBCT and MDCT utilize the varying contrast levels within the body, as the brightness differs between air, fat, bone, tissue, and blood. *Calcification* is defined as a lesion with a threshold above 130 Hounsfield units with an area of three or more contiguous pixels (≥ 1 mm^2). Coronary artery calcium scoring is performed by quantifying coronary calcification throughout the epicardial coronary tree (Fig. 2-2) and is described using either the original Agatston score or the calcium volume score.

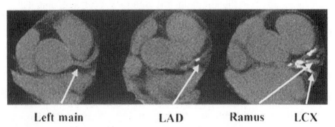

Left main   **LAD**   **Ramus**   **LCX**

FIGURE 2-2. Electron-beam computed tomography with single slice of the heart in three different patients. The ascending aorta, pulmonary artery, left main coronary artery, left anterior descending (LAD) artery, left circumflex (LCX) artery, and ramus intermediate artery are shown. The image on the left demonstrates no coronary artery calcium, the center image demonstrates moderate coronary artery calcification, and the image on the right demonstrates extensive coronary artery calcification. (Adapted from Rumberger JA, Brundage BH, Rader DJ, et al. Electron beam computed tomographic coronary calcium scanning: a review and guidelines for use in asymptomatic persons. *Mayo Clin Proc* 1999;74:243–252, with permission.)

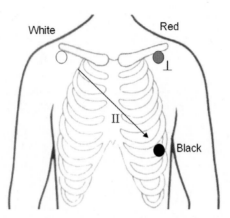

FIGURE 3-1. Standardized electrocardiogram lead placement for performance of cardiac computed tomography. (From Siemens Medical Solutions.)

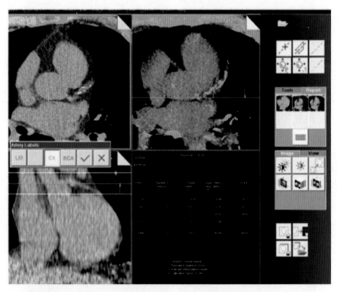

FIGURE 3-6. Screen capture of calcium scoring software. All areas highlighted in color are above the predetermined threshold for calcium. (From Siemens Medical Solutions.)

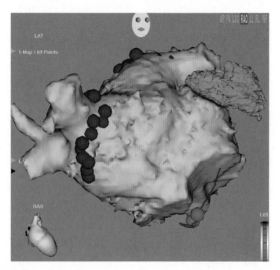

FIGURE 6-2. Carto-Merge and epidural steroid injection fusion.

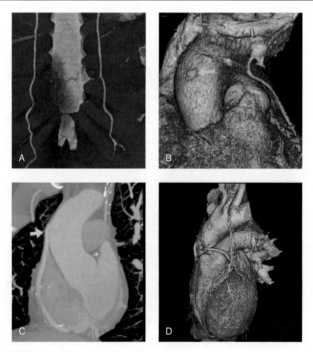

FIGURE 7-1. Computed tomography in coronary artery bypass surgery (CABG). (Reproduced from Topol EJ, Califf RM, et al. Textbook of Cardiovascular Medicine, 3rd Edition. Philadelphia: Lippincott, Williams & Wilkins, 2006.)

The Agatston score is derived from the multiplication of the calcified plaque area and the highest attenuation coefficient. A coefficient value of 1 to 4 is assigned based on the peak Hounsfield units in the plaque (i.e., peak calcium density).[2] This method requires the slice thickness of the scan to be 3 mm and is susceptible to partial volume effects. Subsequently, a more reproducible method to follow the regression and progression of coronary artery calcification was developed by Callister et al.[3] The calcium volume score is independent of calcium density and computes the score based on voxels above the threshold of 130 Hounsfield units.[3] This is an excellent method to track longitudinal changes in coronary calcification; for instance, it can be used as an objective tool to gauge the success of pharmacologic interventions.

INTERPRETATION

Various nomograms exist as the coronary calcium scores differ with age and sex (Table 2-1).[4] Coronary calcification and atherosclerosis increase with age; however, much like the 10-year lag in the development of coronary atherosclerosis in women, the amount of coronary calcium in women is comparable to that in men who are a decade younger. Coronary calcification results in vascular remodeling with varying degrees of luminal impingement and correlates with plaque size. Rumberger et al.[5] demonstrated that quantification of coronary artery calcification is highly correlated with segmental and total coronary artery plaque area ($r = 0.90$, $p < 0.001$ and $r = 0.93$, $p < 0.001$, respectively) in 13 autopsied hearts (Fig. 2.3A and B). The amount of EBCT coronary artery calcification was on average one-fifth of the histopathologic plaque area, on both segmental and total coronary artery tree assessments.[5] This study supported the fact that atherosclerotic plaque is

TABLE 2-1   Coronary Artery Calcium Score Nomogram[a]

	Age (y)							
	35–39	40–44	45–49	50–54	55–59	60–64	65–70
Men (5,433)	(479)	(859)	(1,066)	(1,085)	(853)	(613)	(478)
25th percentile	0	0	0	0	3	14	28
50th percentile	0	0	3	16	41	118	151
75th percentile	2	11	44	101	187	434	569
90th percentile	21	64	176	320	502	804	1,178
Women (4,297)	(288)	(589)	(822)	(903)	(693)	(515)	(485)
25th percentile	0	0	0	0	0	0	0
50th percentile	0	0	0	0	0	4	24
75th percentile	0	0	0	10	33	87	123
90th percentile	4	9	23	66	140	310	362

[a]The number of patients in each group is in parentheses.

Adapted from Raggi P, Callister TQ, Cooil B, et al. Identification of patients at increased risk of first unheralded acute myocardial infarction by electron-beam computed tomography. *Circulation* 2000;101:850–855, with permission.

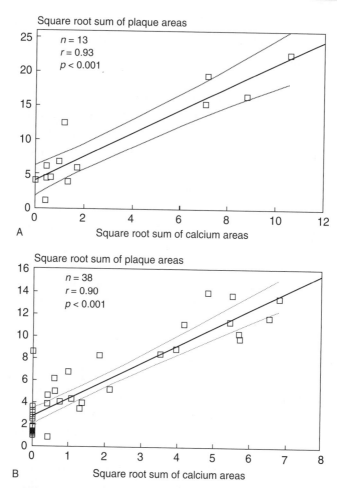

FIGURE 2-3. Relationship between coronary artery calcification on electron-beam computed tomography and plaque area on autopsy hearts, based on the total coronary tree (**A**) and on a segmental model (**B**). (Adapted from Rumberger JA, Simons DB, Fitzpatrick LA, et al. Coronary artery calcium area by electron-beam computed tomography and coronary atherosclerotic plaque area. A histopathologic correlative study. *Circulation* 1995;92:2157–2162, with permission.)

heterogeneous and its composition involves more than just calcium. In addition, not all plaques are made up of calcium, especially the smaller ones.

Accordingly, coronary calcification is specific for coronary atherosclerosis but is not specific for obstructive CAD, as plaque containing calcium can have varying degrees of stenosis and flow limitations. In a study of 1,764 symptomatic patients who were referred for coronary angiography, calcium score assessment with an EBCT scan proved to have high sensitivity and moderate specificity for detecting significant CAD ($\geq$50% stenosis). The coronary calcium score was significantly different between the genders in all age groups; however, the receiver operator curves designate similar accuracy in both genders and age groups. Eleven percent of the men and 22% of the women had a calcium score of 0 and had a very low incidence of significant CAD on conventional angiography (0.7% and 0%, respectively).[6] In the setting of no calcification, the presence of significant CAD is exceedingly rare. In Figure 2-4A and B, one can observe the cutoff values for calcium score based on age for detection of significant and nonsignificant disease, whereas the middle zone indicates an unclear diagnosis.[6] The diagnostic accuracy of EBCT calcium scoring is similar to that of other widely used modalities for assessment of obstructive CAD (Table 2-2).[1] A recent study by Berman et al.[7] established that the most powerful predictor of an ischemic myocardial perfusion study was the presence of coronary calcium. In this study of 1,195 patients, the incidence of an ischemic myocardial perfusion study was very rare (<2%) in patients with a calcium score of <100, while patients with calcium scores of 100 to 399 were in a nebulous zone and it was difficult to predict abnormal stress test results in these patients. In addition, this article revealed that 78% of the patients with a normal stress test result had evidence of varying degrees of coronary artery calcium, thereby affirming the limitation of nuclear stress testing to detect subclinical atherosclerosis. For those

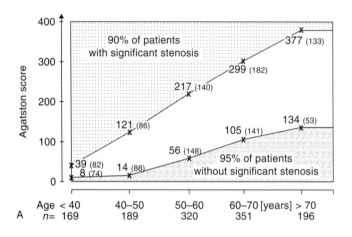

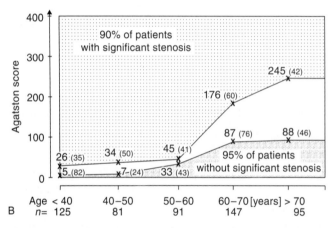

FIGURE 2-4. Calcium score cutoff points for management decisions in men (**A**) and women (**B**) of various age groups. In most patients, obstructive coronary artery disease (CAD) would be likely if the calcium score is above the upper score threshold and unlikely if the calcium score is below the lower score threshold. Calcium scores that fall in the middle zone are imprecise for defining probability of CAD. (Adapted from Haberl R, Becker A, Leber A, et al. Correlation of coronary calcification and angiographically documented stenoses in patients with suspected coronary artery disease: results of 1,764 patients. *J Am Coll Cardiol* 2001;37:451–457, with permission from Elsevier.)

TABLE 2-2 Diagnostic Accuracy of Noninvasive Tests Assessing for Obstructive Coronary Artery Disease

	No. of Patients	Sensitivity (%)	Specificity (%)
Stress treadmill	2,456	52	71
Exercise SPECT	4,480	87	73
Stress echocardiography	2,637	85	77
EBCT calcium	5,730	85	75

SPECT, single photon emission computed tomography; EBCT, electron-beam computed tomography.

Adapted from Budoff MJ, Achenbach S, Blumenthal RS, et al. Assessment of coronary artery disease by cardiac computed tomography: a scientific statement from the American Heart Association Committee on Cardiovascular Imaging and Intervention, Council on Cardiovascular Radiology and Intervention, and Committee on Cardiac Imaging, Council on Clinical Cardiology. *Circulation* 2006;114:1761–1791, with permission.

patients with a calcium score above 100, the number of ischemic stress tests progressively increased as the coronary calcium score increased (Fig. 2-5).[7]

Coronary artery calcium scoring provides prognostic information and aids in early detection and treatment of subclinical atherosclerosis. Many studies have examined the prognostic information in scanning asymptomatic patients. Raggi et al.[4] studied 632 asymptomatic patients who were referred by their physician to undergo an EBCT scan because of CAD risk factors and were followed for 32 months for the occurrence of acute myocardial infarction or cardiac death. All patients were divided into four categories based on their absolute calcium score: zero score, mild score (1–99), moderate score (100–400), and severe score (>400). The annualized cardiac event rate in this cohort progressively increased from the zero score category

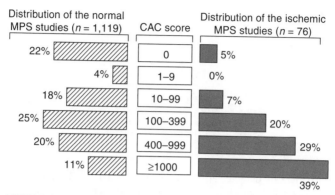

FIGURE 2-5. Distribution of normal and abnormal myocardial perfusion studies with subcategorization based on calcium score. CAC, coronary artery calcium. (Adapted from Berman DS, Wong ND, Gransar H, et al. Relationship between stress-induced myocardial ischemia and atherosclerosis measured by coronary calcium tomography. *J Am Coll Cardiol* 2004;44:923–930, with permission from Elsevier.)

to the severe score category; 0.1% per year in the patients with a calcium score of 0; 2.1% per year in the mild score patients; 4.1% per year in the moderate score patients; 4.8% per year in the severe score patients,[4] as shown in Figure 2-6. These investigators demonstrated that coronary artery calcium scoring adds prognostic information for stratifying patients at risk for cardiac events.

Thereafter, Shaw et al.[8] retrospectively studied 10,377 asymptomatic patients who were referred by their primary care physician for an EBCT scan because of cardiac risk factors. Five-year follow-up data were obtained on the patients, and their Framingham Risk Score was also calculated. Higher calcium scores were associated with an appreciably worse all-cause mortality (Fig. 2-7). Coronary artery calcium score demonstrated superiority to the traditional Framingham Risk Score as

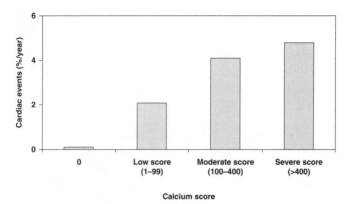

FIGURE 2-6. Coronary artery calcium scores and annual cardiac events. (Adapted from Raggi P, Callister TQ, Cooil B, et al. Identification of patients at increased risk of first unheralded acute myocardial infarction by electron-beam computed tomography. *Circulation* 2000;101:850–855, with permission.)

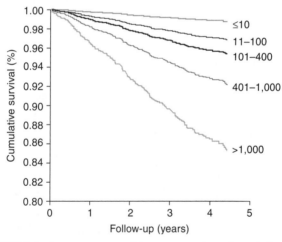

FIGURE 2-7. Coronary artery calcium score and unadjusted all-cause survival. As the baseline calcium score increases the survival rate is worse. (Adapted from Shaw LJ, Raggi P, Schisterman E, et al. Prognostic value of cardiac risk factors and coronary artery calcium screening for all-cause mortality. *Radiology* 2003;228:826–833, with permission from the Radiological Society of North America.)

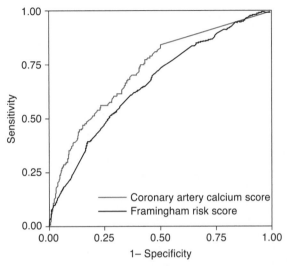

FIGURE 2-8. Receiver operator curves for coronary artery calcium score and Framingham Risk Score. The area under the curve for coronary artery calcium score is larger than the area for Framingham Risk Score ($p < 0.001$). (Adapted from Shaw LJ, Raggi P, Schisterman E, et al. Prognostic value of cardiac risk factors and coronary artery calcium screening for all-cause mortality. *Radiology* 2003;228:826–833, with permission from the Radiological Society of North America.)

the area under the receiver operator curve for coronary artery calcium was significantly greater than that for the Framingham Risk Score (0.73 vs. 0.67, $p < 0.001$; Fig. 2-8). With the progression of Framingham Risk Score, the all-cause mortality increased, and when the patients were further stratified by coronary artery calcium, the all-cause mortality increased with higher coronary artery calcium scores regardless of the Framingham Risk Score (Fig. 2-9).[8]

Many other studies exist regarding EBCT coronary calcium score and risk of CAD. After extensive review of the literature, Rumberger et al.[9] developed guidelines to provide estimates of plaque burden and probability of significant CAD based on

TABLE 2-3 EBCT Calcium Score and Categories of Plaque Burden[a]

EBCT Calcium Score	Plaque Burden	Probability of Significant CAD	Implications for CV Risk	Recommendations
0	No identifiable plaque	Very low, generally <5%	Very low	Reassure patient while discussing general public health guidelines for primary prevention of CV diseases
1–10	Minimal identifiable plaque burden	Very unlikely, <10%	Low	Discuss general public health guidelines for primary prevention of CV diseases
11–100	Definite, at least mild atherosclerotic plaque burden	Mild or minimal coronary stenoses likely	Moderate	Counsel about risk factor modification, strict adherence with NCEP ATP II primary prevention cholesterol guidelines, daily ASA
101–400	Definite, at least moderate atherosclerotic plaque burden	Nonobstructive CAD highly likely, although obstructive disease possible	Moderately high	Institute risk factor modification and secondary prevention NCEP ATP II guidelines. Consider exercise testing for further risk stratification
>400	Extensive atherosclerotic plaque burden	High likelihood (≥90%) of at least one "significant" coronary stenoses	High	Institute very aggressive risk factor modification. Consider exercise or pharmacological test imaging to evaluate for inducible ischemia

EBCT, electron-beam computed tomography; CAD, coronary artery disease; CV, cardiovascular; NCEP ATP II, National Cholesterol Education Program (Adult Treatment Panel II); ASA, acetaminophen.

Adapted from Rumberger JA, Brundage BH, Rader DJ, et al. Electron beam computed tomographic coronary calcium scanning: a review and guidelines for use in asymptomatic persons. *Mayo Clin Proc* 1999;74:243–252, with permission.

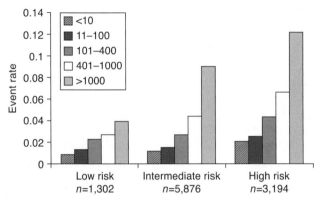

FIGURE 2-9. Distribution of coronary artery calcium scores for each category of Framingham Risk Score. Predicted mortality at 5 years is the event rate. (Adapted from Shaw LJ, Raggi P, Schisterman E, et al. Prognostic value of cardiac risk factors and coronary artery calcium screening for all-cause mortality. *Radiology* 2003;228:826–833, with permission from the Radiological Society of North America.)

the amount of coronary artery calcification (Table 2-3). These guidelines are widely used in the clinical interpretation of coronary artery calcium score imaging tests.

CONCLUSIONS

Calcified plaque is a sensitive tool to detect atherosclerosis but is not specific for identifying obstructive atherosclerosis. High calcium scores are indicative of greater plaque burden and higher risk of coronary events, whereas patients with zero to low calcium scores typically have low coronary events. Identification of coronary artery calcium does not warrant coronary revascularization in asymptomatic patients but provides a rationale for CAD risk factor modification and possibly physiologic assessment of the plaque.

PRACTICAL POINTS

1. Calcification in the coronary arteries can help detect atherosclerosis early in the process, even before the plaque becomes obstructive; therefore, CAD is identified on a CT scan much earlier than it would be on a stress test.

2. Quantification of coronary artery calcification correlates highly with segmental and total coronary artery plaque area.

3. Coronary calcification is specific for coronary atherosclerosis but is not specific for obstructive CAD, as plaque containing calcium can have varying degrees of stenosis and flow limitations.

4. Calcium scoring is not recommended for routine screening, in patients with low or high Framingham risk of heart disease but is useful in those with intermediate risk (Framingham risk score that puts patients at a 10-year risk of 10% to 20% of having a CHD event.)

5. A calcium score >400 in a patient with intermediate risk suggests that the patient may merit from aggressive secondary prevention.

6. A calcium score of 0 is associated with a 96% to 100% probability of no coronary disease, although accuracy is a little less in younger persons.

7. Scans for calcium scoring take only a few minutes, do not require β-blocker administration, and require only a few minutes of the cardiologist's time after the study.

REFERENCES

1. Budoff MJ, Achenbach S, Blumenthal RS, et al. Assessment of coronary artery disease by cardiac computed tomography: a scientific statement from the American Heart Association Committee on Cardiovascular Imaging and Intervention, Council on Cardiovascular Radiology and Intervention, and Committee on Cardiac Imaging, Council on Clinical Cardiology. *Circulation* 2006;114:1761–1791.

2. Agatston AS, Janowitz WR, Hildner FJ, et al. Quantification of coronary artery calcium using ultrafast computed tomography. *J Am Coll Cardiol* 1990;15:827–832.

3. Callister TQ, Cooil B, Raya SP, et al. Coronary artery disease: improved reproducibility of calcium scoring with an electron-beam CT volumetric method. *Radiology* 1998;208:807–814.

4. Raggi P, Callister TQ, Cooil B, et al. Identification of patients at increased risk of first unheralded acute myocardial infarction by electron-beam computed tomography. *Circulation* 2000;101:850–855.

5. Rumberger JA, Simons DB, Fitzpatrick LA, et al. Coronary artery calcium area by electron-beam computed tomography and coronary atherosclerotic plaque area. A histopathologic correlative study. *Circulation* 1995;92:2157–2162.

6. Haberl R, Becker A, Leber A, et al. Correlation of coronary calcification and angiographically documented stenoses in patients with suspected coronary artery disease: results of 1,764 patients. *J Am Coll Cardiol* 2001;37:451–457.

7. Berman DS, Wong ND, Gransar H, et al. Relationship between stress-induced myocardial ischemia and atherosclerosis measured by coronary calcium tomography. *J Am Coll Cardiol* 2004;44:923–930.

8. Shaw LJ, Raggi P, Schisterman E, et al. Prognostic value of cardiac risk factors and coronary artery calcium screening for all-cause mortality. *Radiology* 2003;228:826–833.

9. Rumberger JA, Brundage BH, Rader DJ, et al. Electron beam computed tomographic coronary calcium scanning: a review and guidelines for use in asymptomatic persons. *Mayo Clin Proc* 1999;74:243–252.

CHAPTER 3

How to Perform Cardiac CT Angiography: Dos and Donts

Alex J. Auseon

Proper execution of a cardiovascular computed tomography angiography (CCTA) study actually begins well before the patient's arrival on the day of the scan. The overall objective is a timely, accurate, high-quality procedure performed at minimum risk to the patient. The preceding chapters of this book have focused on procedural indications and the technical aspects of computed tomography (CT). The purpose of this chapter is to provide a practical understanding of the necessary techniques involved in the performance of a typical cardiovascular CT.

PATIENT SELECTION

In order to properly use a diagnostic test to guide therapy, the ordering physician must have an adequate understanding of the test's strengths and shortcomings. In the case of CCTA, its strength lies in excluding obstructive coronary artery disease in the symptomatic, intermediate-risk patient. Its limitations are linked to patient size, volume of coronary artery calcium, heart rate and rhythm, use of iodinated contrast, and exposure to radiation.

With these factors in mind, the true starting point of any scan begins with the patient encounter that results in the physician ordering the test.

Patient obesity presents a significant obstacle to accurate CT imaging. Because the minute size of the typical coronary artery lumen is 2 to 4 mm, achieving submillimeter slice thickness while minimizing the signal-to-noise ratio is paramount. All vendors allow for adjustment of the x-ray tube output in an effort to obtain adequate patient penetration. The majority of scans use a tube voltage of 120 kV, with a range of 80 kV for smaller patients and 140 kV for larger patients. However, each increase results in a subsequent increase in radiation dose without a guarantee of improving the signal-to-noise ratio. Therefore, an arbitrary body mass index threshold of 35 to 40 kg per m^2 has been adopted by centers performing CCTA. If patients exceed this size, other clinical options should be considered, as patient exposure to radiation and contrast may not result in diagnostic-quality images.

When assessing a patient complaining of a chest discomfort syndrome, the physician intuitively calculates the risk of obstructive coronary artery disease as the etiology. For a more objective assessment, use of a well-validated clinical tool is recommended. The Framingham Risk Score is the most commonly employed measure of 10-year cardiovascular risk, allowing patients to be stratified in low-, intermediate-, and high-risk groups. This 10-year risk percentage functions as a surrogate for the likelihood of flow-limiting coronary disease causing anginal symptoms. There are limitations, however, to the Framingham Risk Score, and recent data have led to incorporation of the patient's family history and high-sensitivity

C-reactive protein measurements to produce the Reynolds Risk Score. This tool has also been validated, especially in women, in whom the Framingham Risk Score was not fully representative of true risk. Risk of coronary disease becomes especially important when deciding on ordering a CCTA study, as the presence of large volumes of coronary calcium adversely affect the accuracy of stenosis visualization and quantification. Technical characteristics of CT image formation lead to vessel wall calcium appearing larger in size, resulting in an overestimation of luminal stenoses. In addition, dense calcium may completely obscure visualization of the coronary lumen, even in the absence of flow-limiting obstruction. As a result, patients deemed high risk by Framingham or Reynolds risk scores, or those with high volumes of coronary calcium by prior testing, such as a preceding electron-beam CT, should have their coronary arteries evaluated by means other than CCTA.

POSSIBLE CONTRAINDICATIONS

Diastolic imaging of the coronary arteries, when they are free of motion, requires an imaging modality with a very short temporal resolution, or "shutter speed." It also requires a slow, stable heart rate. Most clinical scanning centers premedicate patients to slow down their heart rate, with agents such as β-blockers or calcium-channel blockers. The most common practice is to either provide a prescription for the patients to take on the morning of the scan or give medication on their arrival. Oral agents can be supplemented with additional intravenous (IV) doses in the final minutes prior to scanning if the heart rate remains elevated (>65–70 beats per minute). *Newer dual-source scanners have improved temporal resolution and thus are less dependent on a heart rate in this specific range.* Patients with frequent ectopy, patients with permanent atrial fibrillation, or those who are unable to lower their heart rates sufficiently despite medication are not good candidates for CCTA.

Use of iodinated contrast should cause significant concern in patients with known risk factors for contrast-induced nephropathy. These include diabetes, hypertension, and pre-existing renal insufficiency. A creatinine clearance rate of <60 mL per minute is considered prohibitive to using iodinated contrast, and therefore to CCTA as well. Strategies to reduce the risk of contrast-induced nephropathy are well detailed in other sources and include IV hydration, with possible additional benefit from oral *n*-acetylcysteine. In addition, patients need to be rigorously screened for intolerance and allergic reactions to iodinated contrast. Each scanning center should have specific protocols to instruct patients when premedicating those who are allergic, as well as to deal with emergent issues of anaphylactoid responses.

Exposure to radiation during CCTA has been the subject of investigation and concern since its inception. First and foremost, any patient believed to be pregnant should always undergo confirmatory urine testing to prevent fetal exposure. *The dose of radiation received during a single scan is 10 to 20 mSv, depending on parameters of each individual protocol and use of dose-modulation techniques. It is roughly comparable to a nuclear stress perfusion study and believed to be two to three times that of a typical diagnostic catheterization.* This will not be discussed in detail but should factor into patient selection in the context of younger patients, potential subsequent diagnostic imaging exposure, and risk of malignancy.

PATIENT ARRIVAL AT THE SCANNING CENTER

On the day prior to their CCTA study, patients should be contacted and told to fast for approximately 4 hours and avoid caffeine on the day of their procedure. They should be instructed about the sequence of events that will be part of the center's scanning protocol and should be assessed in a holding area. At that time vitals can be documented, especially heart rate and blood pressure, so decisions about heart rate–lowering medications can be made. A large-bore IV line, no smaller than 20 gauge, should be placed, preferably in the right antecubital vein.

ADMINISTRATION OF HEART RATE–LOWERING MEDICATION

Patients should be again screened for contraindications, allergies, and intolerances to medications, especially β-blockers, during their initial assessment. If there are no issues, patients should be given an oral dose of 50 to 100 mg metoprolol, preferably 30 to 60 minutes before their scan. Calcium channel blockers, primarily verapamil, serve as a useful alternative when patients are unable to tolerate β-blockade. In addition to heart rate, frequent premature atrial or ventricular contractions can also change the interval between each cardiac cycle, interfering with accurate electrocardiogram (ECG) gating and leading to nondiagnostic images. Occasionally, a single IV dose of lidocaine can be used to suppress frequent ectopy and allow for a stable heart rate. As mentioned earlier, the common heart rate goal is 60 to 70 beats per minute for 16- and 64-slice scanners, with newer dual-source machines allowing accurate imaging at higher rates.

PROPER ELECTROCARDIOGRAM GATING

Because image acquisition relies on ECG gating, a reliable signal is imperative. Standard practice should include cleaning the skin with alcohol and an abrading agent. Men should

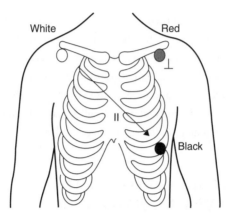

FIGURE 3-1. Standardized electrocardiogram lead placement for performance of cardiac computed tomography. (From Siemens Medical Solutions.) (See color insert.)

be shaved at the electrode sites if hair interferes. Proper placement of electrodes is in a standard formation (Fig. 3-1), with all three being placed outside of the desired field of view. Every effort, including replacing or repositioning suboptimal leads and trying all lead configurations, should be made to provide a consistent ECG tracing. The scanner housing has an ECG readout above the center of the gantry, allowing the heart rate and rhythm to be seen from all areas of the scanning suite (Figs. 3-2 and 3-3).

PATIENT POSITIONING

Today's CT scanners have the ability to scan with the patient entering the gantry either feet first or head first. At our institution, they are placed in a supine position with their feet nearest to the scanner. To ensure comfort, a pillow, knee rest, and blankets should be used, as patient discomfort may lead to movement, corrupting image quality. Most vendors employ use of a laser

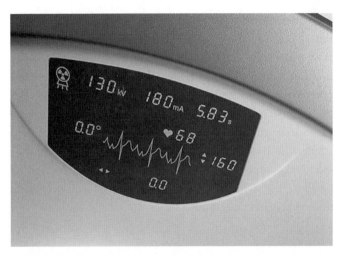

FIGURE 3-2. Electrocardiogram panel on the front of the scanner housing. (From Siemens Medical Solutions.)

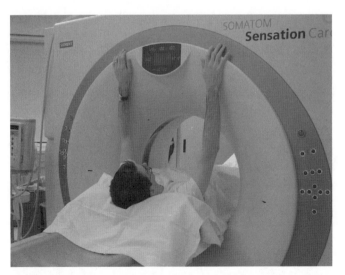

FIGURE 3-3. Patient position within the scanner (feet-first position). *Note:* both arms extended upward along the housing, allowing for more complete and rapid flow during power injection of contrast dye and saline into the right antecubital vein.

sight that allows proper vertical table height. The horizontal line should run along the mid- to anterior axillary line when the patient's arm is raised. When the patient is in the optimal position to begin, he or she will be midway through the scanner, crossing through the gantry approximately at the level of the diaphragm (Fig. 3-3). The arm containing the antecubital IV (usually the right) should be extended upward and held straight, in part to allow for unobstructed venous flow during rapid contrast injection. In the case of a feet-first scanning position, the right hand can also rest on the gantry housing prior to starting table motion.

FINAL STEPS BEFORE INITIATING THE SCANNING PROCEDURE

At this point, the patient is nearly ready to begin undergoing the CCTA. *In order to fully ensure the highest quality data during the short image acquisition time, the scanning technologist should help the patient rehearse holding their breath for the anticipated duration of time required for scanning.* The length of a typical scan varies, lasting from 8 to 16 seconds, depending on the size of the field of view (FOV) included in the desired image. A rehearsed breath hold allows the technologist to learn the behavior of the patient's heart rate in addition to the length of time the patient can tolerate holding the breath effectively. A significant number of patients perform a breath hold against a closed epiglottis, essentially performing a Valsalva maneuver, which may significantly alter the heart rate. In most instances, this is an advantageous phenomenon, allowing a longer motion-free period to obtain images of the coronary arteries during diastole. However, it may take more than one cardiac cycle for this to manifest, leading to the technologist choosing to initiate the subsequent scanning procedure after a few seconds' delay, instead of directly at the beginning of the breath hold period.

The patient should also be fully informed about the expected effects of rapid contrast injection into the antecubital IV site. Common sensations include a sensation of warmth, altered temperature, discomfort at the site, and intolerance or allergy symptoms, such as nausea or itching. The last step before initiating the scanning procedure is to give a single dose of sublingual nitroglycerin, either in tablet form or in spray form, to fully dilate the coronary bed and increase the ability to clearly visualize distal branches. Contra-indications to nitroglycerin such as patients on sildenafil should be obtained, as this interaction could potentially lead to harm.

SCANNING PROCEDURE

A full CCTA is a multistep process with specific steps that vary by scanning vendor. The basic overall sequence, however, is somewhat conserved despite differences in equipment, software, and terminology. Once the patient is in place with a satisfactory heart rate, the technologist and/or physician take their seat at the scanning workstation (Fig. 3-4).

CHEST TOPOGRAM

In order to choose an FOV for image acquisition, the first step in the process is to obtain a chest topogram. The patient moves quickly through the scanner, receiving a low-radiation, noncontrast scan analogous to a chest x-ray. The resultant image, displayed on the technologist's workstation, allows for a targeted scanning border to be selected (Fig. 3-5). The perimeter should range from the level of the carina to 1 cm below the diaphragm, a distance of approximately 12 to 14 cm, in patients undergoing a standard examination to exclude coronary disease. In those patients with

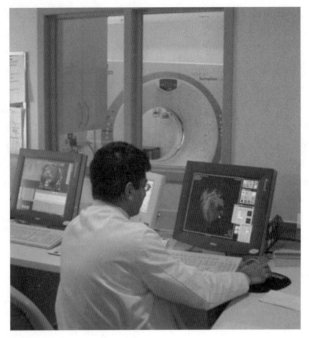

FIGURE 3-4. Scanner workstation.

previous bypass surgery and a left internal mammary artery grafted to the left anterior descending, the FOV should be expanded to include the upper lung fields, thereby capturing the branch point off the left subclavian artery. These additional data require more time to acquire and substantially increase the number of seconds the patient needs to hold their breath during scanning.

CALCIUM SCORING

A second low-radiation (0.7–3 mSv), noncontrast scan moves the patient through the gantry again, this time undergoing a calcium scoring acquisition. The full, selected FOV is included

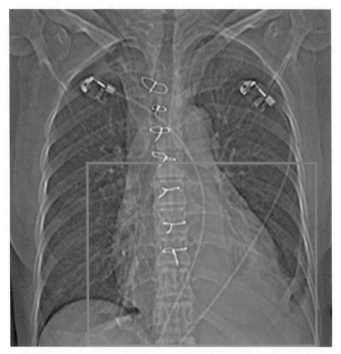

FIGURE 3-5. Chest topogram. Border indicates the volume to be scanned. (From Siemens Medical Solutions.)

in the data set and is designed to highlight any calcification, including extracardiac structures (Fig. 3-6). The technologist should routinely take a moment at this point to scroll through the full volume of data and qualitatively assess coronary calcium burden before proceeding to the next step. If a patient is found to have even a moderate amount of coronary calcium in only one territory, consideration should be given to aborting the remaining portion of the scan. The specific rationale for this lies in balancing radiation and contrast exposure against the value of a nondiagnostic scan. If a large amount of coronary calcium prevents accurate visualization of the vessel lumen,

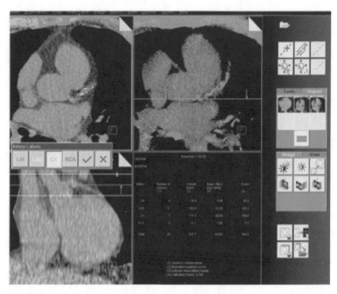

FIGURE 3-6. Screen capture of calcium scoring software. All areas highlighted in color are above the predetermined threshold for calcium. (From Siemens Medical Solutions.) (See color insert.)

then the patient has been negatively exposed without gaining useful information about the patient's health. If necessary, the technologist can also quickly use the workstation's software to calculate a calcium score. While there is no specific number that would prompt a physician to cancel the contrast portion of a scan, it would be reasonable to consider cancellation in any patient with a score of 500 or greater (either Agatston or volumetric), especially in a single-vessel territory.

CONTRAST INJECTION AND CORONARY ANGIOGRAPHY

Most scanners have clear prompting on their workstation monitors during scanning steps, allowing straightforward transition from one portion to the next. The final phase requires the patient to hold their breath for their previously described time of image acquisition. A prerecorded voice command will commonly instruct the patient to hold still and not breathe. During the scan time, the IV contrast injection takes place, opacifying the coronary arteries.

Proper execution of CCTA involves precise synchronization of image acquisition with the patient's ECG tracing and the IV injection of a contrast bolus. Too early, and contrast has not had time to reach the left heart. Too late, and only the descending aorta is adequately opacified. To achieve the necessary monophasic peak of contrast enhancement, a dual-head power injector is used, with iodinated contrast in one cartridge and a saline chaser in the other. Injection is timed by one of the two methods: a *test bolus* or *automatic bolus tracking*. For both, a region of interest is first highlighted in the ascending aorta at the level of the pulmonary artery bifurcation (Fig. 3-7). With the test bolus strategy, a small bolus is injected (20 mL at 4–5 mL per second) with an accompanying saline chaser of similar volume. The chosen slice is repeatedly imaged every 2 seconds until contrast is seen passing through the region. These data are then analyzed using workstation software to plot a graph illustrating the delay in seconds before full enhancement in the aorta and coronary arteries. This specific delay is then factored into the manual timing needed to follow the start of imaging after contrast injection.

Automatic bolus tracking begins identically after opening the software package, with a region of interest chosen in the same position in the ascending aorta. A predetermined threshold of Hounsfield units is chosen before the scan, allowing the software to scan the slice every 2 seconds after injection. When the computer senses that the signal intensity

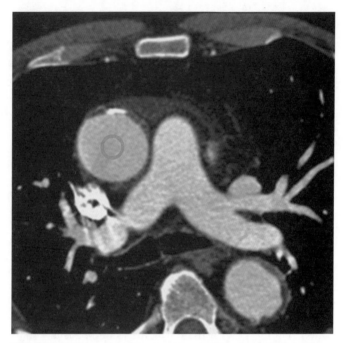

FIGURE 3-7. Region of interest selected within the ascending aorta. Signal intensity will rise after rapid injection of intravenous contrast. The time to peak can be calculated during observation of a test bolus injection. With automatic bolus tracking, the computer will initiate the full angiographic scan protocol once the intensity has risen above the predetermined Hounsfield unit preset. (From Siemens Medical Solutions.)

inside the region of interest has risen above the threshold (typically 100–120 Hounsfield unit), the full 0.6-mm thickness volume is scanned automatically. Both methods are equally effective, with advantages and disadvantages. Test bolus injection allows the patient to experience the sensation of injection before undergoing the full diagnostic

TABLE 3-1	Scanner Parameters for Multistep Cardiac CT Protocol[a]	
Coronary calcium scoring		
kV		120
Effective mAs		310
Slice width (mm)		3
Slice collimation (mm)		1.2
Pitch		0.2
Kernel		B30f
Coronary CT angiography		
kV		120
Effective mAs		700–900
Detector collimation (mm)		0.6
Slice thickness (mm)		0.75
Pitch		0.2
Rotation time (s)		0.33
Reconstruction interval (mm)		0.5
Kernel		B30f

kV, kilovolt; mAs, milliamperes; CT, computed tomography.
[a]Specifically for 64-slice CT scanner.

portion of the scan, lowering anxiety and potentially heart rate as well. Automatic bolus detection is easy to execute and removes much of the human error that might lead to a nondiagnostic scan.

Once the patient finishes the breath hold and injection phase, the scan is finished. The IV and ECG leads can now be removed and properly discarded. The patients should be led to a patient recovery room, where they can get dressed, undergo final assessment of their vital signs and be screened for any unexpected contrast reactions. There is no specified time

TABLE 3-2	Patient Selection, Preparation, and Premedication

Screen for relative contraindications to CCTA
  Body mass index of >35–40 kg/m^2
  High risk of vessel wall calcium from coronary artery disease
  Inability to lower heart rate to <70 bpm with medication
  Irregular heart rhythm
  Risk factors for contrast-induced nephropathy

Key points in patient preparation on the day of scanning
  NPO for 4 h
  No caffeine
  Large-bore IV (at least 20 gauge) in right antecubital vein
  Ensure adequate skin contact with ECG leads
  Patient instruction and breath hold rehearsal

Patient Premedication
  Obtain baseline heart rate and blood pressure
  100 mg metoprolol PO if HR is >75 bpm 30 min prior to scan
  50 mg metoprolol PO if HR is 65–75 bpm 30 min prior to scan
  Additional IV doses of 5 mg metoprolol if HR is still >70 bpm just prior
    to scan
  Sublingual nitroglycerin, either 0.4 mg tablet or single spray just prior
    to scan

CCTA, cardiovascular computed tomography angiography; bpm, beats per
  minute; NPO, non per os (nothing by mouth); IV, intravenous;
  ECG, electrocardiogram; PO, per os (by mouth); HR, heart rate.

duration before it is deemed safe for them to leave the imaging
facility, and this is up to each institution's discretion.

PRACTICAL POINTS

1. The strength of coronary CT lies in excluding
   obstructive coronary artery disease in the symptomatic, intermediate-risk patient.

2. The limitations of coronary CT are related to patient size, volume of coronary artery calcium, heart rate and rhythm, use of iodinated contrast, and exposure to radiation.

3. If patients exceed the body mass index threshold of 35 to 40 kg per m^2, other clinical options should be considered, as patient exposure to radiation and contrast may not result in diagnostic-quality images.

4. Patients deemed high risk by Framingham or Reynolds risk scores, or those with high volumes of coronary calcium by prior testing, such as a preceding electron-beam CT, should have their coronary arteries evaluated by means other than CCTA.

5. Patients with frequent ectopy, permanent atrial fibrillation, or those who are unable to lower their heart rate sufficiently despite medication are not good candidates for CCTA.

6. The dose of radiation received during a single scan is 10 to 20 mSv, depending on parameters of each individual scan and use of dose-modulation techniques. It is roughly comparable to a nuclear stress perfusion study and believed to be two to three times that of a typical diagnostic catheterization.

7. β-Blockers are usually used to maintain the heart rate between 60 and 70 beats per minute.

8. Although there is no specific number that would prompt a physician to cancel the contrast portion of a scan, it would be reasonable to consider cancellation in any patient with a calcium score of 500 or greater (either Agatston or volumetric), especially in a single-vessel territory.

ADDITIONAL READING

1. Halliburton SS, Abbara S. Practical tips and tricks in cardiovascular computed tomography: patient preparation for optimization of cardiovascular CT data acquisition. *J Cardiovasc CT* 2007;1: 62–65.
2. Pannu HK, Alvarez W Jr, Fishman EK. β-Blockers for cardiac CT: a primer for the radiologist. *AJR* 2006;186:S341–S345.
3. Decramer I, Vanhoenacker PK, Sarno G, et al. Effects of sublingual nitroglycerin on coronary lumen diameter and number of visualized septal branches on 64-MDCT angiography. *AJR* 2008; 190:219–225.
4. Lin EC. Coronary computed tomography angiography: principles of contrast material administration. *J Cardiovasc CT* 2007;1: 162–165.
5. Budoff M, Achenbach S, Blumenthal RS, et al. Assessment of coronary artery disease by cardiac computed tomography: a scientific statement from the American Heart Association Committee on Cardiovascular Imaging and Intervention, Council on Cardiovascular Radiology and Intervention, and Committee on Cardiac Imaging, Council on Clinical Cardiology. *Circulation* 2006;114:1761–1791.

An Interventional Cardiologist's Perspective on Coronary CT Angiography

Ernest Mazzaferri

INTRODUCTION

Cardiovascular disease (CVD) accounts for approximately 1 out of every 2.8 deaths in the United States each year, or approximately 2,400 deaths per day equaling one death every 36 seconds. CVD claims more lives every year in the United States than cancer, chronic lower respiratory disorders, diabetes mellitus, and accidents combined.[1] In 2004, approximately 1,471,000 inpatient cardiac catheterizations were performed and the estimated direct and indirect cost of CVD in the United States was $151.6 billion for the year 2007.[2] Understandably, the diagnosis and prevention of CVD in a cost-effective manner is critically important to the welfare of patients and the economic survival of the health care system.

THE DIAGNOSIS OF CORONARY ARTERY DISEASE: CONVENTIONAL CORONARY ANGIOGRAPHY

Conventional coronary angiography (CCA) has long been considered the gold standard for the diagnosis of coronary artery disease (CAD), with greater than 50% luminal narrowing of a coronary artery considered evidence of significant CAD. However, CCA is not without limitations. It is an invasive procedure with radiation exposure that incurs a certain level of risk to the patient depending on the experience of the operator as well as the patient's clinical condition, coronary anatomy, and comorbidities. While the general risk of having a major complication from diagnostic CCA is low (Table 4-1), if a complication occurs to a patient, the complication rate is 100%. Therefore, despite the fact that CCA remains the gold standard for

TABLE 4-1	Risk of Cardiac Catheterization ($n = 59,792$)
Mortality (%)	0.11
Myocardial infarction (%)	0.05
Cerbrovascular accident (%)	0.07
Arrhythmia (%)	0.38
Vascular complication (%)	0.43
Contrast reaction (%)	0.37
Hemodynamic compromise (%)	0.26
Perforation of a heart chamber (%)	0.28
Other (%)	0.28
Total (%)	1.7

Reprinted from Noto TJ Jr, Johnson LW, Krone R, et al. Cardiac catheterization 1990: a report of the Registry of the Society for Cardiac Angiography and Interventions (SCA&I). *Cathet Cardiovasc Diagn* 1991;24:75, with permission from John Wiley & Sons, Inc.

identifying CAD, an abundance of resources have been allocated for the development and integration of noninvasive studies in an effort to keep patients out of the cardiac catheterization lab.

THE DIAGNOSIS OF CORONARY ARTERY DISEASE: CORONARY COMPUTED TOMOGRAPHY ANGIOGRAPHY

Coronary computed tomography angiography (CCTA) is gaining popularity as a diagnostic test of choice for the determination of the presence and severity of CAD. As opposed to noninvasive functional studies that infer coronary artery stenosis, CCTA is the only noninvasive study that provides structural and anatomic information similar to that provided by CCA, albeit without the risk of an invasive approach. Nonetheless, the risk of radiation exposure and intravenous contrast exposure remains.

The development of CCTA has been through much iteration, culminating in the 64-slice scanners. The most significant improvement that the 64-slice scanner has over the smaller array scanners (40-slice or less) is the ability to perform a complete scan of the heart, or a specific area of interest, in a much shorter time,[3] yet there is also improvement in spatial resolution.[4] In groundwork investigations involving small numbers of patients, CCTA has been a remarkably sensitive tool with an excellent negative predictive value (Table 4-2), supporting its stance as a tool to rule out significant CAD. The negative predictive value of CCTA in most studies has been above 98%, excluding patients in whom interpretation was insufficient for a variety of reasons. It has been suggested that when referral to CCA is questionable, CCTA may identify patients with normal angiograms and potentially decrease the number of invasive procedures performed.

TABLE 4-2	Accuracy of 16-Slice and 64-Slice CCTA				
16-Slice CT	**N**	**Sensitivity (%)**	**Specificity (%)**	**NPV (%)**	**Unevaluable (%)**
Nieman	59	95	86	97	7
Ropers	77	93	92	97	12
Kuettner	58	98[a]	98[a]	100[a]	—
Mollet	128	92	95	98	—
Martuscelli	64	89	98	98	16
Fine	50	87	97	98	2
Kaiser	149	30	91	83	23
Aviram	22	86	98	98	—
Hoffmann	33	89[b]	95[b]	97[b]	—
Kuettner	124	85	98	96	7
Mollet	51	95	98	99	—
Morgan-Hughes	58	89[c]	98[c]	98[c]	—
Schujif	45	98	97	100	6
Hoffmann	103	95	98	99	6
Achenbach	50	94	96	99	4
64-Slice CT					
Leschka	53	94	97	99	—
Raff	70	86	95	98	12
Leber	59	88[b]	97[b]	99[b]	—
Mollet	52	99	95	99	2
Ropers	82	95	93	99	4
Fine	66	95	96	95	6

CCTA, coronary computed tomography angiography; CT, computed tomography; NPV, negative predictive value.

[a]Analysis in all patients with Agatston score <1,000.

[b]Per-segment analysis, proximal and mid segments.

[c]Analysis in all 36 patients with an Agatston score <400.

Adapted from Hendel RC and the CCT/CMR Writing Group. ACCF/ACR/SCCT/SCMR/ASNC/NASCI/SCAI/SIR Appropriateness Criteria for Cardiac Computed Tomography and Cardiac Magnetic Resonance Imaging—Online Appendix.

Conversely, in the largest randomized trial evaluating the diagnostic accuracy of CCTA (64-scanner) compared with that of CCA ($N = 316$), CCTA had a 91% positive predictive value and an 83% negative predictive value.[5] Importantly, the patient population studied was asymptomatic, had suspected CAD, and was scheduled for CCA. Interestingly, out of the 405 patients recruited for this trial, 89 were excluded because they had coronary artery calcium scores above 600 and another 21 were excluded for technical reasons (110 of 405, 27%). Therefore, more than a quarter of the patients were ultimately excluded from the denominator and not included in the accuracy calculations. Furthermore, there was not a good correlation between the anatomic location of disease between CCTA and CCA, demonstrating the former as an unreliable method to define the coronary segment requiring revascularization.[5]

SPECIAL PATIENT POPULATIONS

The value of CCTA seems to be better in certain specified patient populations. There is evidence to suggest that CCTA is an excellent tool in the evaluation for patency of coronary artery bypass grafts as well as for the evaluation of the origin and pathway of anomalous coronary arteries.

The perceived advantage in imaging coronary bypass conduits is due to the lack of motion artifact and often large caliber of the conduit vessel. In a report of 138 consecutive patients with a total of 418 arterial and venous bypass conduits, 64-slice CCTA had both a sensitivity and a specificity of 97%.[6] The clinical application of these data continues to be uncertain as it is equally important to evaluate the native coronary arteries in symptomatic patients with prior bypass surgery, and with this endeavor the sensitivity and specificity of CCTA drops significantly.[7] Ultimately, unless the goal is to exclusively evaluate the patency of the bypass grafts, the definitive study continues to be CCA.

It is well known that the risk of sudden cardiac death is increased in patients with anomalous coronary origins, specifically when the proximal segment of an anomalous coronary artery courses between the aorta and the pulmonary artery. While most invasive cardiologists are familiar with well-described CCA techniques such as the "dot and eye" method[8] to identify the course and origin of anomalous coronary arteries, it is relatively safe to say that a good number of invasive cardiologists are not completely confident in their own application and interpretation of the technique. CCTA, therefore, provides an excellent alternative for the evaluation of anomalous coronary arteries (Clinical Vignette; Figs. 4-1 and 4-2A–C).

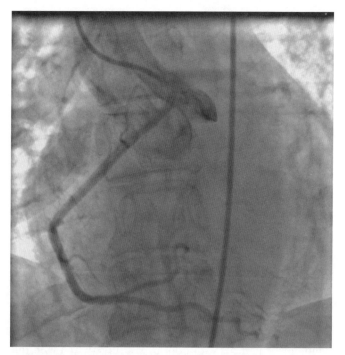

FIGURE 4-1. Catheter angiography of the right coronary artery shows origin from the left sinus of Valsalva. The left coronary artery is also visible because of the reflux of contrast from the injection. Ao, aortic root. (Courtesy of Raymond D. Magorien, MD, FACC, The Ohio State University.)

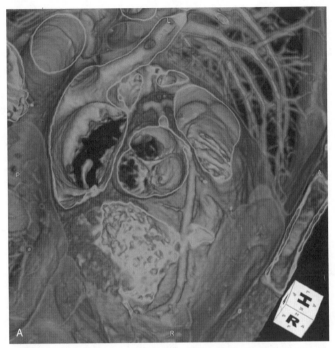

FIGURE 4-2. A: Volume rendered computed tomography angiography data with contrast-filled lumen subtracted in this figure shows the normal caliber left coronary ostium compared to the slit-like orifice of the right coronary artery, which regains normal caliber on exiting the narrow space between the aorta and the right ventricular outflow tract. The aortic sinuses are labeled as follows: L, left; R, right; and N, noncoronary. Volume rendering with the contrast-filled lumen appearing bright shows the larger caliber of the proximal right coronary artery (*arrowhead*) during diastole (**B**) compared with systole (**C**). Ao, aortic root; LA, left atrium. (*Continued*)

While the number of studies and patients are limited, the potential efficacy of CCTA in the identification of the origin and course of anomalous coronary arteries was demonstrated in a study of 17 patients referred for evaluation after CCA and echocardiography yielded equivocal findings. Of these patients,

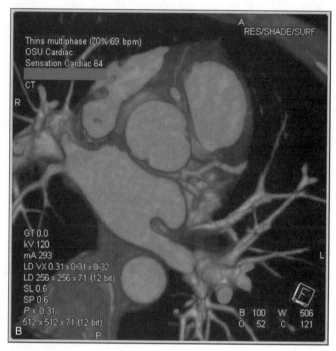

FIGURE 4-2. *Continued*

CCTA accurately identified the origin and course of all 20 anomalous coronary arteries that were in question by CCA and echocardiography.[9] Cardiac magnetic resonance angiogram is also a valuable tool in imaging anomalous coronary arteries and may be a more practical option in some patients because of the lack of radiation needed to acquire images.

OTHER POTENTIAL UTILIZATIONS

There are several areas of interest in the future clinical uses of CCTA. Some studies are designed to help avoid CCA altogether, others to assist where CCA has failed, and those designed

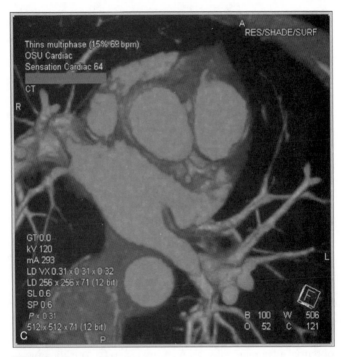

FIGURE 4-2. *Continued*

to assist the planning of percutaneous coronary intervention (PCI).

To establish whether CCTA can guide the decision whether or not to use CCA in patients with symptoms suggestive of CAD and intermediate-risk myocardial perfusion imaging (1%–3% annual event rate), Danciu et al.[10] retrospectively evaluated 421 patients. The findings reveal that in this specific patient population, CCTA can identify up to 80% of patients at low risk for events in whom CCA can be safely avoided. In these low-risk patients, there was a 0.3% (1 in 343) rate of combined end-point of death, myocardial infarction, and revascularization compared with 72% (55 of 76) in the overall group referred for CCA.

The success rate of PCI in patients with chronic total occlusion (CTO) is relatively low, and CCTA may be helpful in determining which patients may benefit from an attempt at percutaneous revascularization. If the *trans*-luminal calcium burden of the CTO is ≥50% via CCTA, it has been shown to be an independent predictor of failed PCI.[11] Other unique applications that require further investigation involve the assessment of ostial coronary artery lesions, bifurcation stenoses, and in-stent restenosis.

A UNIQUE PERSPECTIVE ON PLAQUE MORPHOLOGY

Angina typically results from coronary artery stenosis greater than 70%; thereby vessels with lesser stenosis usually remain asymptomatic. Paradoxically, it is well known that ST-elevation myocardial infarction is often the result of a ruptured plaque with less than 50% stenosis.[12,13] One of the potential advantages of CCTA compared to CCA is the unique ability to directly visualize and quantify the amount of plaque in the vessel lumen.[14,15] Like many other areas of advancing biomedical technologies, this capability precedes robust clinical data on how this may apply to current patient care.

Supportively, Hoffman et al.[16] evaluated the differences between culprit lesions in acute coronary syndromes (ACS) and stable lesions in patients with ACS or stable angina ($N = 37$). It was identified that culprit lesions in patients with ACS had a significantly greater plaque area and a higher remodeling index than the stable lesions in patients with ACS (or stable angina). While further investigation is forthcoming, the prospect of identifying patients at risk for acute coronary syndrome is an exciting endeavor. This advancement may also offer the opportunity to monitor progression of disease and evaluate the response of atheromatous plaque to medical therapy.

COST-EFFECTIVENESS

Over the last 5 years, the rapid evolution and improvement of CCTA and CT calcium scoring in the detection of coronary atherosclerosis has led to widespread use of the technology in broadened clinical populations despite a lack of clear scientific evidence. The Medicare Payment Advisory Commission (MPAC) reported to Congress in March 2007 that CT imaging had the highest rate of growth (14.7%) of all cardiovascular services in 2004–2005, with an estimated cost of $100 billion during that time.[17] Because of this growing demand for CT imaging, Congress expressed mounting concern about the potential contribution of cardiac imaging to the overall increase in societal health care costs.

This concern led to a Science Advisory Statement issued by the American Heart Association supporting the following principles[18]:

1. Imaging studies should be performed by physicians who meet published standards of training and experience from medical societies accredited by the Accreditation Council for Graduate Medical Education.

2. These procedures should be performed in high-quality laboratories with appropriate facilities and technical personnel who are adequately trained in imaging procedures and related safety standards.

Despite this proclamation, it is estimated that approximately 1,000 or more 64-slice CT scanners are now operational in the United States, with approximately 100 to 200 having staffs with the experience and reading skills needed to replicate the results of clinical trial data.[19]

Using a decision tree model submitting hypothetical cohorts of patients with different pretest likelihoods for CAD, Dewey and Hamm[20] compared the cost-effectiveness of recent approaches (coronary angiography and calcium scoring using

TABLE 4-3	Pretest Likelihood Calculation for CAD					
	Typical Angina[a] (%)		Atypical Angina[b] (%)		Nonanginal Chest Pain[c] (%)	
Age (y)	Women	Men	Women	Men	Women	Men
30–49	26	70	4	22	1	5
40–49	55	87	13	46	3	14
50–59	79	92	32	59	8	22
60–69	91	94	54	67	19	28

CAD, coronary artery disease.

[a]All three characteristics of angina pectoris present (retro-sternal location, triggered by exercise, and release during rest or after nitroglycerin).

[b]Only two of the above-mentioned characteristics are present.

[c]Only one of the above-mentioned characteristics is present.

According to Diamond GA, Forrester JS. Analysis of probability as an aid in the clinical diagnosis of coronary-artery disease. N Engl J Med 1979;300:1350–1358.

Adapted from Dewey M, Hamm B. Cost effectiveness of coronary angiography and calcium scoring using CT and stress MRI for diagnosis of coronary artery disease. Eur Radiol 2007;17:1301–1309.

CT and stress magnetic resonance imaging) to the diagnosis of CAD with those of traditional diagnostic modalities (conventional angiography, exercise ECG, and stress echocardiography). This model has several significant limitations; however, it was concluded that up to a pretest likelihood of 50% for CAD (Table 4-3), CCTA is the most cost-effective procedure, being superior to the other new and most commonly used traditional modalities. With a higher likelihood of disease (pretest probability above 60%), CCA is the most cost-effective procedure. While this model is far from perfect, it provides a glimpse into the future as to how CCTA may fit into the diagnostic armamentarium of CAD.

RISKS

One of the dangers of a noninvasive test is that the risks of the procedure are often unintentionally de-emphasized by physicians and poorly understood by the patients. There are two key direct potential risks from CCTA that need to be considered when evaluating a patient for this study.

1. *Radiation exposure*: The radiation exposure during CCTA is generally between 7 and 21 mSv versus approximately 2 to 6 mSv from conventional diagnostic angiography.[21,22] In comparison, the average radiation from a head CT is 1 to 2 mSv and from a diagnostic chest x-ray is 0.04 to 0.06 mSv. A single screening with a CCTA in a 45-year-old adult would impart a lifetime attributable cancer mortality risk of 0.08% (1 in 1,250), while 30 annual screens would impart a lifetime attributable cancer mortality risk of 1.9% (about 1 in 50).[23] In contrast, screening mammography has about 100-fold less radiation exposure than that from screening CCTA.[24]

2. *Contrast exposure*: Generally, 60 to 120 cm^3 of iodinated contrast is delivered during CCTA. This is roughly equivalent to the contrast delivered during CCA. The risk of an allergic reaction to iodinated contrast remains, as does the risk of nephrotoxicity, especially in patients with chronic renal insufficiency or diabetes mellitus.

There are other potential risks of CCTA that warrant consideration, including the potential risk of β-blocker administration (in certain patient populations) as a target heart rate of 60 to 70 beats per minute is needed for diagnostic accuracy. Also, not to be minimized is the indirect potential risk caused by a false-positive or false-negative study.

TABLE 4-4	ACC-F Appropriateness Criteria for CCTA

Indication	Appropriateness Criteria
Symptomatic evaluation of chest pain syndrome in patient with intermediate pretest probability of CAD *and* an uninterpretable ECG or unable to exercise	A
Symptomatic evaluation of acute chest pain syndrome in patient with intermediate pretest probability of CAD *and* no ECG changes *and* negative cardiac enzymes	A
Evaluation of chest pain syndrome with uninterpretable or equivocal stress test result	A
Evaluation of coronary arteries in patient with new-onset heart failure to assess etiology	A
Evaluation of suspected coronary anomalies	A
Symptomatic evaluation of chest pain syndrome in patient with high pretest probability of CAD	I
Symptomatic evaluation of acute chest pain syndrome in patient with high pretest probability of CAD *and* ST-segment elevation and/or positive cardiac enzymes	I
Evaluation of chest pain syndrome with evidence of moderate to severe ischemia on stress test (exercise, perfusion, or stress echo)	I
Asymptomatic evaluation of patient with low *or* moderate CHD risk (Framingham risk criteria)	I
Asymptomatic evaluation of patient with high CHD risk (Framingham) *and* prior calcium score ≥400 (or within 2 years prior CCTA or CCA without significant obstructive disease)	I
Asymptomatic evaluation of bypass grafts and coronary anatomy	I
Asymptomatic evaluation for in-stent restenosis and coronary anatomy after PCI	I

ACC-F: American College of Cardiology Foundation; CCTA, coronary computed tomography angiography; CAD, coronary artery disease; ECG, electrocardiogram; A, appropriate; I, inappropriate; CHD, coronary hear disease; CCA, conventional coronary angiography; PCI, percutaneous coronary intervention.
Adapted from Hendel RC, et al. Appropriateness criteria for CCT/CMR. *JACC* 2006;48(7):1475–1497.

PRACTICAL USE AND CURRENT RECOMMENDATIONS

As few clinical practice guidelines currently exist for the role of CCTA, under the auspices of the American College of Cardiology Foundation, an appropriateness review was conducted and published.[25] Several clinical scenarios were deemed appropriate and inappropriate for CCTA (Table 4-4).

SUMMARY

CCTA is a rapidly advancing technology and has made such significant strides over the last decade, which has been propelled from the research arena to the day-to-day care of patients. It has progressed from the bulky 4-slice CT system to the efficient 64-slice CT system, and the development of flat-plate technology is on the horizon. Although still emerging, the current technology dictates that over the next decade CCTA will be a major competitor in cardiovascular imaging. Until randomized trial data catch up to this advanced technology, it is likely that CCTA will only increase the volume of diagnostic CCA.

CLINICAL VIGNETTE

Courtesy of Subha V. Raman

A 49-year-old woman without relevant medical history presented to her physician with complaints of exertional chest tightness radiating to shoulders and neck. Physical examination was unremarkable. Electrocardiography demonstrated sinus rhythm with inferior and anterolateral T-wave abnormalities. Stress nuclear imaging suggested a small region of distal anterior wall ischemia. Cardiac catheterization showed an anomalous origin of a large dominant right coronary artery (RCA) from the left sinus of Valsalva (Fig. 4-1). To better define the origin and proximal course of the anomalous coronary artery, she was referred for cardiac computed tomography (CTA). The 64-slice CTA examination confirmed the anomalous origin of the RCA while also delineating an interarterial course between the aorta and the right ventricular outflow tract (Fig. 4-2). She then underwent single-vessel coronary artery bypass grafting with a right internal mammary artery graft to the distal right coronary artery. Subsequent stress testing was within normal limits, and she has remained symptom-free at 5-month follow-up.

PRACTICAL POINTS

1. Negative 64-slice CT study is reliable in excluding significant CAD.
2. The finding of stenosis on 64-slice CT usually requires confirmation.
3. The presence of a high pretest probability of CAD strengthens the diagnosis when stenosis is detected by 64-slice CT.
4. The sensitivity and specificity of 64-slice CT ranges from 86% to 93% and 96%, respectively.
5. Calcification within the coronary arteries can result in false-negative and, more commonly, false-positive findings concerning the presence of coronary stenosis. Therefore, calcification of the coronary artery segments makes them not assessable by CT.
6. Coronary lumen is generally not well seen in the region of a coronary stent.

REFERENCES

1. Minino AM, Heron MP, Smith BL. Deaths: preliminary data for 2004. *Natl Vital Stat Rep.* 2006;54:1–49.
2. Rosamond W, Flegal K, Friday G, et al. Heart disease and stroke statistics—2007 update. *Circulation* 2007;115:e69–e161.
3. Schussler JM. An interventionalist's perspective: diagnosis of cardiovascular disease by CT imaging. In: Budoff MJ, Shinbane JS, eds. *Cardiac CT Imaging: Diagnosis of Cardiovascular Disease.* London: Springer Verlag; 2006:147–163.
4. Pugliese F, et al. Diagnostic accuracy of non-invasive 64-slice CT coronary angiography in patients with stable angina pectoris. *Eur Radiol* 2006;16:575–582.
5. Miller JM. Data from CORE-64 Trial. *AHA Scientific Sessions Presentation, November 2007.*
6. Meyer TS, et al. Improved non-invasive assessment of coronary artery bypass grafts with 64-slice computed tomographic angiography in an unselected patient population. *J Am Coll Cardiol* 2007 Mar 6;49(9):946–950.
7. Ropers D, et al. Diagnostic accuracy of non-invasive angiography in patients after bypass surgery using 64-slice spiral computed tomography with 330-ms gantry rotation. *Circulation* 2006 Nov 28;114(22):2334–2341.
8. Serota H, et al. Rapid identification of the course of anomalous coronary arteries in adults: the "dot and eye" method. *Am J Cardiol* 1990;65:891–898.
9. Datta J, et al. Anomalous coronary arteries in adults: depiction at multi-detector row CT-angiography. *Radiology* 2005 Jun;235(3):812–818.
10. Danciu SC, et al. Usefulness of multislice computed tomographic coronary angiography to identify patients with abnormal myocardial perfusion stress in whom diagnostic catheterization may be safely avoided. *Am J Cardiol* 2007;100:1605–1608.
11. Soon KH, et al. CT coronary angiography predicts the outcome of percutaneous coronary intervention of chronic total occlusion. *J Interven Cardiol* 2007;20:359–366.
12. Little WC, et al. Can coronary angiography predict the site of a subsequent myocardial infarction in patients with mild-to-moderate coronary artery disease? *Circulation* 1988 Nov;78(5 Pt 1):1157–1166.

13. Giroud D, et al. Relation of the site of acute myocardial infarction to the most severe coronary arterial stenosis at prior angiography. *Am J Cardiol* 1992 Mar 15;69(8):729–732.

14. Achenbach S, et al. Detection of calcified and noncalcified coronary atherosclerotic plaque by contrast-enhanced, submillimeter multidetector spiral computed tomography: a segment-based comparison with intravascular ultrasound. *Circulation* 2004;109(1):14–17.

15. Fuster V, et al. Atherothrombosis and high-risk plaque. Part II: approaches by noninvasive computed tomographic/magnetic resonance imaging. *J Am Coll Cardiol* 2005 Oct 4;46(7):1209–1218.

16. Hoffmann U, et al. Noninvasive assessment of plaque morphology and composition in culprit and stable lesions in acute coronary syndrome and stable lesions in stable angina by multidetector computed tomography. *J Am Coll Cardiol.* 2006 Apr 18; 47(8):1655–1662. Epub 2006 Mar 27.

17. Medicare Payment Advisory Commission. *Report to the Congress: Medicare Payment Policy.* March 2005.

18. Gibbons RJ, Eckel RH, Jacobs AK. AHA science advisory: the utilization of cardiac imaging. *Circulation* 2006;113:1715–1716.

19. Miller JM. Interview. *Cardiology News.* 2007 Dec;(5):12.

20. Dewey M, Hamm B. Cost effectiveness of coronary angiography and calcium scoring using CT and stress MRI for diagnosis of coronary artery disease. *Eur Radiol* (2007)17:1301–1309.

21. Chartrand-Lefebvre C, et al. Coronary computed tomography angiography: overview of technical aspects, current concepts, and perspectives. *JACR* 2007 Apr;58(2):91–109.

22. Morin RL, et al. Radiation dose in computed tomography of the heart. *Circulation* 2003 Feb 18;107(6):917–922.

23. Brenner DJ, Elliston CD. Estimated radiation risks potentially associated with full-body CT screening. *Radiology* 2004;232: 735–738.

24. Black WC, Czum JM. Screening coronary CT angiography: no time soon. *J Am Coll Radiol* 2007 May;4(5):295–299.

25. Hendel RC, et al. Appropriateness criteria for CCT/CMR. *JACC* 2006 Oct 3;48(7):1475–1497.

CHAPTER 5

CT Angiography of the Peripheral Arteries: The Interventionalist's Perspective

Quinn Capers IV

The cardiovascular interventionalist has a very pragmatic view of imaging: he requires a blueprint with which to plan procedures. That blueprint, or map, should be accurate, with no surprises for the operator. It should be detailed, providing information such as the location and origin of collateral vessels, the presence and relative amounts of calcium, the adequacy of the "runoff," etc. Finally, the results of the imaging study should be reproducible, so that the operator can follow interventional results longitudinally. The accuracy, reproducibility, and level of detail provided by various vascular imaging studies can be affected by patient-related factors and factors particular to the type of study.

Tomographic imaging techniques provide three-dimensional views of the arterial lumen and wall. Such images are superior to the "luminogram" provided by conventional angiography for interventional planning. For example, a heavily calcified atheroma that protrudes anteriorly from the posterior aspect of the vascular wall may require that the directional atherectomy device be directed "away from" the operator during the procedure to ensure maximal debulking. Likewise, the presence of mural thrombus proximal and distal to a complex atherosclerotic stenosis is best treated with placement of a long vascular stent to provide a scaffold and minimize embolization. In these scenarios, a two-dimensional silhouette of the lumen would be inadequate to optimize results and patient safety. As a result, for many vascular interventionalists, tomographic techniques have become the preferred imaging modalities for pre-interventional planning.

Three techniques are currently available for three-dimensional, tomographic imaging of the blood vessel: intravascular ultrasound, magnetic resonance angiography (MRA), and computed tomographic angiography (CTA). Other modalities are currently being investigated, such as optical coherence tomography. Table 5-1 compares intravascular ultrasound, MRA, and CTA and their utility for the interventionalist. Intravascular

TABLE 5-1	Comparison of IVUS, MRA, and CTA and their Utility for the Interventionalist		
	IVUS	**MRA**	**CTA**
Invasive/Noninvasive	Invasive	Noninvasive	Noninvasive
Radiation exposure?	No	No	Yes
Iodinated contrast?	No	No	Yes
Useful with severe Ca^{2+}?	Yes	No	$+/-$
Useful in presence of stainless steel stents?	Yes	No	Yes
Useful in advanced renal failure?	Yes	Yes, without contrast	No

IVUS, intravascular ultrasound; MRA, magnetic resonance angiography; CTA, computed tomographic angiography.

ultrasound is extremely useful as an adjunct to catheter-based vascular interventions and has been shown to improve long-term outcomes of interventional procedures in the peripheral circulation.[1,2] However, since arterial puncture is necessary to employ this procedure, its use is generally reserved for patients in whom the decision to intervene has already been affirmed. Because both CTA and MRA are noninvasive techniques, the threshold for their use is lower, and they are used more widely as screening tools.

MRA generates images based on energy released when atoms are exposed to a powerful magnetic field. When compared to invasive digital subtraction angiography (DSA), MRA has been shown to be sensitive and specific for the detection of severe stenoses in the carotid, aortic, upper extremity, and lower extremity circulations. The lack of radiation exposure to the patient is an advantage for MRA, as is the lack of necessity for iodinated contrast. This latter fact makes MRA imaging particularly useful in patients with renal impairment. It has been recently discovered that the devastating illness nephrogenic systemic fibrosis can complicate the use of gadolinium-based contrast agents in patients with a severe diminution of creatinine clearance.[3] Thus, clinicians must be cautious about ordering contrast-enhanced MRA studies in persons with advanced renal failure. The benefits and limitations of MRA are compared to those of CTA in Table 5-2.

CTA, like MRA, is very useful in the evaluation of the vascular disease patient and complements the limitations of the latter. MRA is not useful in imaging arterial segments previously treated with stainless steel stents because of metal artifacts. In contrast, CTA can adequately visualize stents and the lumen within the stent in most cases. Raza et al.[4] found that CTA was comparable to the gold standard DSA in the detection of in-stent restenosis in renal arteries. A recent *in vitro* study found that CTA is slightly superior to MRA in differentiating between

TABLE 5-2	**MRA versus CTA**

MRA
    Benefit
        Noninvasive
        No iodinated contrast
        Able to image wall as well as lumen
    Limitations
        Unable to use in patients with pacemaker/defibrillator
        Images limited in cases of severe calcification
        Not useful in arterial segments with stainless steel stents
CTA
    Benefit
        Noninvasive
        Able to image wall as well as lumen
        Useful in patients with pacemaker/defibrillator
        Useful in patients with stainless steel stents
        Useful in patients with severe vascular calcification
    Limitations
        Radiation exposure necessary
        Iodinated contrast necessary

MRA, magnetic resonance angiography; CTA, computed tomographic angiography.

severe in-stent stenoses and occlusions in both stainless steel and nitinol stents.[5] Although contemporary success rates at opening short segment total occlusions are high, differentiating between severely stenosed and totally occluded target lesions is extremely important. Choice of equipment, adjunctive use of antithrombotic or fibrinolytic agents, and even counseling the patient as to the likelihood of success are all potentially affected by the preoperative knowledge of whether the in-stent lesion is a total occlusion.

Heavy calcification in arterial walls and atherosclerotic plaques remains a technical challenge to the cardiovascular interventionalist. Not only does calcium thwart the interventionalist at the lesion by decreasing lesion compliance and making the plaque relatively resistant to compression, cutting, or "drilling," but a heavily calcified artery can frustrate attempts to advance interventional equipment to the lesion as well. When considering a focal left popliteal artery stenosis contralateral to the accessed femoral artery, a strategy of advancing equipment "up and over" the aortoiliac bifurcation is associated with fewer complications than an antegrade left femoral artery puncture. However, severe calcification of the aortic bifurcation and left iliofemoral arterial segment can impede advancement of sheaths, wires, and stents to the target lesion. These problems can be effectively addressed by choosing tapered, "kink"-resistant sheaths, sheaths and wires coated with hydrophilic polymers, and stiff wires with very flexible tips. Thus, preoperative knowledge of the extent of calcium is useful for selecting equipment that will optimize chances for success. Imaging of severely calcified lesions remains a challenge for both MRA and CTA. However, computed tomography (CT) imaging is quite effective for the detection of calcium proximal and distal to the lesion as well as within the lesion of interest, although lesion topography may be obscured. Such imaging would be adequate, however, to inform the operator of the extent and location of calcium.

The presence of collateral circulation to the end-organ is a tell-tale sign of lesion chronicity and can adversely impact the likelihood of a successful revascularization procedure, as in the case of a total occlusion when a large collateral vessel originates from the corner of a blunt total occlusion. In such a case, preferential advancement of the guidewire into the collateral vessel rather than the lumen of the target vessel is problematic. However, although an unfortunately oriented collateral can serve as a "foe," collateral circulation to a severely ischemic limb can be the interventionalist's best "friend" in the event of an unsuccessful revascularization attempt. In a patient with critical limb ischemia, a large collateral vessel arising near the proximal edge of a total occlusion may be the patient's last source of distal limb perfusion. The loss of such an important structure during an attempted percutaneous procedure, due to dissection, plaque shift, or as a consequence of stent placement is unfortunate, and is to be avoided at all cost. A preoperative imaging procedure that can reliably identify collateral vessels is very useful for the interventionalist. CTA of the lower extremity vessels has been shown to be nearly as accurate as DSA in detecting and locating collateral circulation and superior to DSA in delineating vessels below the ankle.[6]

Since many vascular interventionalists will follow their postoperative patients periodically, they will need serial imaging studies to complement the clinical examination. CTA is attractive as a candidate imaging study to follow the postoperative vascular patient. In fact, CTA is widely considered the gold standard for follow-up of patients after endovascular repair of abdominal aortic aneurysms (EVAR) and is particularly useful for detecting endoleaks in the years following EVAR. Follow-up of the renal and iliac stent patient has also been performed successfully with CTA, though arterial Doppler and duplex studies are used for this purpose more often at our institution. The risk of radiation-induced cancer is not negligible with serial CTA procedures,[7] and although new technology is being introduced that will lower the radiation dose to patients undergoing CTA, this concern will likely limit the use of CTA as a serial-imaging procedure to follow vascular patients.

A recent study compared CTA with DSA in the assessment of peripheral vascular disease.[8] In 50 consecutive patients, 21 vascular segments were defined in each leg and compared with DSA with regard to length, severity of stenosis, and number of lesions. They found that mean sensitivity and specificity in the detection of significant stenosis (>70%) were 100% and 99.5% in iliac arteries, 97.4% and 99.0% in femoro-popliteal arteries, and 98.3% and 99.8% in the infrapopiliteal arteries, respectively.

There was high agreement between CTA and DSA for exact stenosis severity, length of lesion, and number of lesions in this study as shown by high κ values ranging from 0.7 to 1.0 for each parameter. These findings suggest that CTA is an accurate tool for assessing peripheral vascular disease.

In summary, the vascular interventionalist has several options for preoperative, noninvasive vascular studies with which to guide his therapeutic procedures. CTA is reproducible, useful in cases of heavily calcified arteries, and able to accurately diagnose in-stent stenoses. Limitations of this technique include the necessity for radiation exposure and the use of iodinated contrast agents. However, CTA has rapidly become a very useful tool in the diagnosis and management of vascular disease, and future enhancements are likely to improve on its limitations. The collaborative nature of the discipline of vascular intervention welcomes the vascular imaging specialist as a vital partner on the vascular team.

PRACTICAL POINTS

1. CTA is accurate in detection of stenosis severity, number, and length of lesions.[8]
2. CTA was comparable to the gold standard DSA in the detection of in-stent restenosis in renal arteries.
3. CTA of the lower extremity vessels has been shown to be nearly as accurate as DSA in detecting and locating collateral circulation and superior to DSA in delineating vessels below the ankle.
4. CTA is widely considered the gold standard for follow-up of patients after EVAR and is particularly useful for detecting endoleaks in the years following EVAR.
5. Limitations of this technique include the necessity for radiation exposure and the use of iodinated contrast agents.

REFERENCES

1. Buckley CH, Arko FR, Lee S, et al. Intravascular ultrasound scanning improves long-term patency of iliac lesions treated with balloon angioplasty and primary stenting. *J Vasc Surg* 2002;35: 316–323.

2. Navarro F, Sllivan TM, Bacharach JM. Intravascular ultrasound assessment of iliac stent procedures. *J Endovasc Ther* 2000;7: 315–319.

3. Sadowski EA, Bennet LK, Chan MR, et al. Nephrogenic systemic fibrosis: risk factors and incidence estimation. *Radiology* 2007 Apr;243(1):148–157.

4. Raza SA, Chughtai AR, Wahba M, et al. Multislice CT angiography in renal artery stent evaluation: prospective comparison with intra-arterial digital subtraction angiography. *Cardiovasc Interv Radiol* 2004 Jan/Feb;27(1):9–15.

5. Blum MR, Schmook M, Shcernthaner R, et al. Quantification and detectability of in-stent stenosis with CT angiography and magnetic resonance angiography in arterial stents in vitro. *Am J Roentgenol* 2007 Nov;189(5):1238–1242.

6. Albrecht T, Foert E, Holtkamp R, et al. 16 MDCT angiography of aortoiliac and lower extremity arteries: comparison with digital subtraction angiography. *Am J Roentgenol* 2007 Sep;189(3): 702–711.

7. Einstein AJ, Herzlova MJ, Rajagopalan S. Estimated risk of cancer associated with radiation exposure from 64-slice computed tomography coronary angiography. *JAMA* 2007 Jul 18;298(3): 317–323.

8. Scherntkhaner R, Stadler A, Lomoschitz F, et al. Multidetector CT angiography in the assessment of peripheral occlusive disease: accuracy in detecting the severity, number and length of stenoses. *Eur Radiol* 2008;18:665–671.

6

An Electrophysiologist's Perspective of Cardiac CT

Raul Weiss and Subha V. Raman

The focus of this chapter is to provide the readers with a practical and up-to-date review of the clinical uses of cardiac computed tomography (CT) in patients with electrophysiological disorders.

Cardiac imaging can be accomplished by multiple modalities, such as transthoracic echocardiogram, transeophageal echocardiogram, cardiac magnetic resonance imaging, cardiac catheterization, and nuclear imaging. These different modalities are usually complementary to each other. Appropriate cardiac imaging selection is usually dictated by the suspected underlying pathology: body habitus of the patient, presence of esophageal disorders, renal insufficiency, presence of implantable devices, and age of the patient.

Cardiac CT is useful in patients with electrophysiology disorders because it provides fine detail of anatomic structures, and it can be used in patients with previously implanted pacemakers, internal cardiac defibrillators (ICDs), or implantable loop recorders. Cardiac CT is not operator dependent like other cardiac imaging modalities, and software can reconstruct three-dimensional images as well. Newer systems can be mounted in the electrophysiology laboratory and the CT scan can be performed immediately prior to or during the electrophysiological procedure.

In the past decade, the field of clinical cardiac electrophysiology has seen an exponential increase in the number and complexity of procedures performed. The areas of greater advancements are in the treatment of atrial fibrillation, sudden cardiac death prevention, and device-based treatment for congestive heart failure, with the use of either biventricular pacemakers or biventricular pacemakers/defibrillators.

These advancements were made possible because of a series of breakthroughs in each of the earlier mentioned areas:

- In the area of atrial fibrillation, the description from Haissaguerre et al.[1,2] demonstrated that premature atrial contraction originating from the pulmonary veins can trigger atrial fibrillation. This same group reported[1–3] pulmonary vein isolation by using radiofrequency ablation and targeting the muscle sleeve that connects the vein "electrically" to the left atrium and potentially cure atrial fibrillation.

- In the area of sudden cardiac death prevention, multiple large randomized clinical trials have shown mortality benefit. Patients with aborted sudden cardiac death (secondary prevention) and patients with ventricular function <36% (primary prevention) have been shown to have improved survival rates with ICD implantation.

- In the area of congestive heart failure, multiple studies have shown that resynchronization devices improve congestive heart failure symptoms, quality of life, and survival; decrease the number of hospitalizations, B-type natriuretic peptide, epinephrine, and noerepinephrine levels, and mitral regurgitation; and increase dP/dT (not at the expense of increase oxygen consumption).

A CT image plays a crucial role in the treatment of atrial fibrillation; it serves as a road map to where the radiofrequency ablative procedure will take place.

CT imaging helps delineate the anatomy of the coronary sinus and its tributary. It can assist in making an *a priori* selection of a lateral or posterolateral branch to be targeted during transvenous implantation. Also, the lack of target vessels in the desired area may prevent the patient from having an unnecessary transvenous attempt. This allows the patient to proceed directly to an epicardial implantation.

Finally, cardiac CT can readily identify high-risk groups for sudden cardiac death, such as patients with low ejection fraction.

The most common applications of cardiac CT to the field of electrophysiology can be divided into two broad categories.

1. Delineation of the cardiac anatomy prior to an electrophysiological intervention.
   a. Left atrium, left atrial appendage, and pulmonary veins anatomy to guide atrial fibrillation ablation.
   b. Evaluation of the coronary sinus and its branches prior to left ventricular (LV) lead implantation.
   c. Evaluation prior to Wolff–Parkinson–White syndrome (WPW) ablation (Ebstein's anomaly).
   d. Evaluation of the anatomy in patients with congenital heart disease or surgically corrected congenital heart disease prior to delineating the ablative procedure.
2. Risk assessment of sudden cardiac death.
   a. Evaluation of the ejection fraction in ischemic and nonischemic myopathies.
   b. Evaluation of congenital heart disease.

DELINEATION OF THE CARDIAC ANATOMY PRIOR TO AN ELECTROPHYSIOLOGICAL INTERVENTION

LEFT ATRIUM, LEFT ATRIAL APPENDAGE, AND PULMONARY VEINS ANATOMY TO GUIDE ATRIAL FIBRILLATION ABLATION

The management of atrial fibrillation consists basically of anticoagulation and rate or rhythm control. Anticoagulation is indicated in a group of patients at risk for thromboembolic event.[4,5]

Rate control is usually reserved for patients with mild symptoms, or those who are asymptomatic, or those in whom antiarrhythmics are contraindicated. Rate control can be achieved either pharmacologically or by applying radiofrequency ablation to the atrioventricular node and implantation of a pacemaker.

Rhythm control, conventionally performed by suppressing atrial fibrillation with antiarrhythmic drugs, has yielded disappointing results. There have been reported suppression rates of only up to 60% at 1 year after sinus rhythm was restored.

In 1998, Haissaguerre et al.[2] in a landmark work reported that pulmonary vein ectopy can initiate atrial fibrillation. The same group reported that atrial fibrillation can be "cured" in 75% to 80% of patients by electrical isolation of the pulmonary veins, applying radiofrequency ablation in the "muscle sleeve" connecting the pulmonary veins with the left atrium. With the encouraging results of catheter-based ablation and the disappointing results of medical management, the paradigm of treatment radically changed from a suppression of the arrhythmia with antiarrhythmics drugs to a curative approach with a catheter-based approach.

Deep knowledge of the atrial anatomy is crucial for procedural success and minimization of complications. This procedure heavily relies on reconstruction of the atrial anatomy. The size of the left atrium and the type of atrial fibrillation[6,7] usually dictate the type of ablative approach. In patients with a large left atrium, wide areas of circumferential lesions around pulmonary veins and connecting lines are often performed (Fig. 6-1).

It also should be noted that the advancements in the ablative treatment of atrial fibrillation parallel the advancements in mapping systems, catheter technologies, and to a certain extent robotic navigation. Newer mapping systems are capable

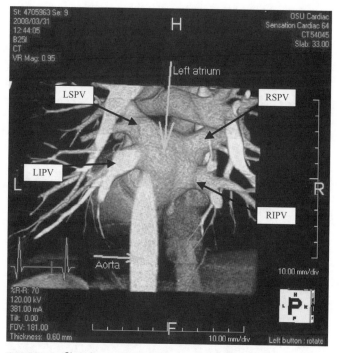

FIGURE 6-1. Showing normal pulmonary veins, left atrial appendage, and relationship of the left atrium and the esophagus.

of incorporating anatomical data with electrophysiological recording, creating a true electro-anatomical three-dimensional chamber. The most commonly used mapping systems with capability to import CT imaging into a real-time map are Carto-Merge (Biosense Webster) (Fig. 6-2) and EnSite 3000® (Endocardial Solutions, St Jude Medical) (Fig. 6-2). Electro-anatomical mapping allows for precise deployment of the radiofrequency lesions. These systems are essential for lesion-tracking after they have been deployed.

With the advent of this procedure, complications such as atrial esophageal fistula or phrenic nerve paralysis can be explained by the proximity of these structures to the left atrium and pulmonary veins. Intuitively, avoidance of energy delivered in the close proximity of these areas may prevent these complications.

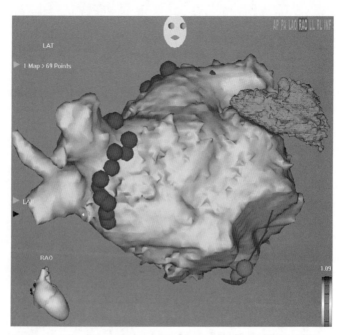

FIGURE 6-2. Carto-Merge and epidural steroid injection fusion. (See color insert.)

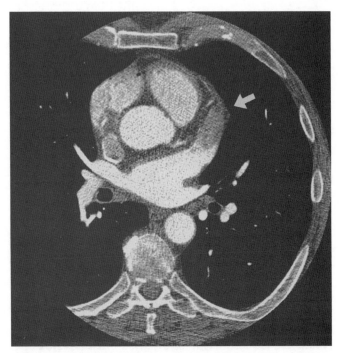

FIGURE 6-3. Filling defect consistent with thrombus in the left atrial appendage in a patient in atrial fibrillation. (Reproduced from Topol EJ, Califf RM, et al. Textbook of Cardiovascular Medicine, 3rd Edition. Philadelphia: Lippincott Williams & Wilkins, 2006.)

Cardiac CT also provides evidence of left atrial appendage clot (Fig. 6-3). The evaluation of left atrial appendage clot has being performed mainly with a transesophageal echocardiogram. It will be a significant advantage for patients' comfort (as well as a decrease in procedural cost) if a single test can be performed to evaluate the pulmonary vein, assess the left atrial size, and rule out left atrial appendage clot.

Cardiac CT has also been shown to be a sensitive test in the diagnosis of pulmonary vein stenosis and in the follow-up of patients in whom a pulmonary vein intervention was performed because of the high re-stenosis rate (Fig. 6-4).

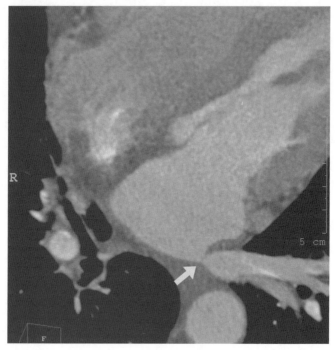

FIGURE 6-4. Pulmonary vein stenosis 6 months after radiofrequency ablation for atrial fibrillation in a 63-year-old patient with progressive exertional dyspnea. (Reproduced from Topol EJ, Califf RM, et al. Textbook of Cardiovascular Medicine, 3rd Edition. Philadelphia: Lippincott Williams & Wilkins, 2006.)

EVALUATION OF THE CORONARY SINUS AND ITS BRANCHES PRIOR TO LEFT VENTRICULAR LEAD IMPLANTATION

Resynchronization therapy is accomplished by synchronizing right and left ventricular pacing to the atrial activity (in patients with normal sinus rhythm). It is indicated in patients with congestive heart failure, New York Heart Association classes 3 and 4, ejection fraction of ≤0.35, left bundle branch block, and a

QRS duration of more than 120 ms, not responding to medical therapy.[8]

Implantation of an LV lead for resynchronization therapy can be achieved by a transvenous or thoracotomy approach. The advantage of a transvenous approach is the relative simplicity of the procedure, a shorter length of stay, and increased longevity of the leads. Other advantages of the transvenous approach are that it is performed under local anesthesia, without the need for intubation, which reduces overall complications for this fragile group of patients.[9] The disadvantages of this approach are the fact that the leads can be positioned only where an epicardial vein is present, which may not be the ideal position for pacing. One clear advantage of the surgical approach is the use of electrode design for epicardial implantation, which face the myocardium and are unlikely to be associated with phrenic nerve stimulation, a complication reported to be as high as 4% in clinical trials with a transvenous approach.

Lateral and posterolateral branches of the coronary venous anatomy have been shown to be the most beneficial location for pacing. These locations have shown the greatest hemodynamic improvement. The knowledge that those branches are well developed and of a certain diameter will likely be associated with a successful implant.

The Thebesian valve is the valve that covers the inferior and posterior aspect of the coronary sinus ostium, which is well developed in up to 30% of the cases and can make the implantation of the LV lead difficult by impeding the cannulation of the coronary sinus. The CT scan can also assess the take off of the coronary sinus when high cannulation may be difficult.

The valve of Vieussens represents the end of the great cardiac vein and the beginning of the coronary sinus. This valve is competent in approximately 20% of the cases. The valve of Vieussens can impede advancement of the LV lead into the lateral branches. Externally, the valve of Vieussens is marked by a smaller diameter external ring. The vein of Marshall (or ligament of Marshall when is not patent) drains into the confluence of great cardiac vein and coronary sinus. In a small number of implants, this valve may impede lead advancement. These valves may require venoplasty for successful LV lead implant.

Evaluation of the size of the right atrium is also important. The right atrium serves as a "working station" for the telescopic sheaths that will deliver the coronary sinus lead. A large right atrium signifies a need for far-reach delivery systems and large curve catheters. It may also predict a difficult coronary sinus cannulation.

Persistent left superior vena cava can be identified with cardiac CT, and implantation of the device from the right axillary vein approach would be advisable.

EVALUATION PRIOR TO WOLFF–PARKINSON–WHITE SYNDROME ABLATION (EBSTEIN'S ANOMALY)

In a small percentage of cases, patients with WPW are associated with Ebstein's anomaly. CT scan can identify the ventricular displacement of the tricuspid valve and atrialization of the right ventricle in these patients. Evaluation of Ebstein's anomaly in patients with WPW, although feasible, is not commonly used. Echocardiography is the preferred method because it is readily available and is without the inherent risk of radiation.

CT scan has the advantage of being able to detect coronary sinus diverticula, a saclike formation with a ventricular extension that originates within the first centimeter or two from the coronary sinus ostium. Posteroseptal accessory pathways can be ablated from within this structure.

RISK ASSESSMENT OF SUDDEN CARDIAC DEATH

EVALUATION OF THE EJECTION FRACTION IN ISCHEMIC AND NONISCHEMIC MYOPATHIES

Multiple studies have shown the superiority of ICDs in preventing sudden cardiac death in high-risk patients. Sudden cardiac death prevention can be primary if the patient had not had a previous event, or can be secondary in patients with aborted sudden cardiac death or ventricular tachycardia with hypotension or syncope (Fig. 6-5).

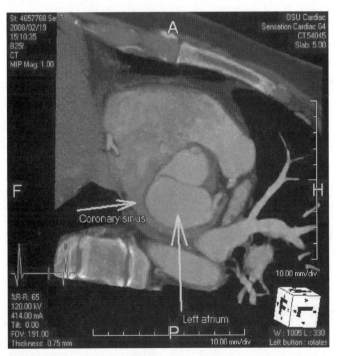

FIGURE 6-5. Normal coronary sinus and tributaries in two views.

The first group of patients who showed benefit from ICD therapy was the patients with prior myocardial infarction, LV function ≤40%, nonsustained ventricular tachycardia, and a positive electrophysiological study that cannot be suppressed with procainamide infusion. This was the first study that showed mortality benefit. The benefit was also substantial with a reduction of 54% in all-cause death. This was a primary prevention study.[10]

Antiarrhythmic Versus Implantable Defibrillators (AVID), a secondary prevention trial, also showed a mortality benefit of approximately 30% at 3 years in patients with ICD.[12]

The largest randomized trial of primary prevention of sudden cardiac death was reported in 2005. Two thousand five hundred patients with an ejection fraction of ≤35% and ischemic and nonischemic myopathy New York Heart Association classes 2 and 3 were included. Once again there was a significant mortality benefit in the ICD group.[12]

CT scan can identify patients at high risk for sudden cardiac death by accurate measurement of the LV function. Three-dimensional reconstruction of CT angiography can directly visualize coronary arteries, which may point out the etiology of the myopathy process.

Cardiac CT does not play a significant role in the evaluation of right ventricular cardiomyopathy, hypertrophic cardiomyopathy, or infiltrative disease of the heart. Cardiac magnetic resonance has largely replaced cardiac computed tomography for these indications.

EVALUATION OF CONGENITAL HEART DISEASE

Multiple congenital malformations, either surgically corrected or not, may progress to LV dysfunction and can be associated with sudden cardiac death. Three-dimensional reconstruction of the anatomy and scar density can be assessed accurately by this technique.

The presence of normal myocardium between scar tissue and anatomical structures serves as substrate for atrial or ventricular arrhythmias. Atrial and ventricular arrhythmias can cause hemodynamic compromise in this population. Persistent supraventricular arrhythmia can lead to tachycardia-induced myopathy and ventricular arrhythmia can lead to sudden cardiac death.[13]

PRACTICAL POINTS

1. Radiofrequency ablation of atrial fibrillation is the most common electrophysiologic indication for multidetector computed tomography (MDCT), although it is also utilized in the ablation of other arrhythmias. MDCT is useful in that it
   - provides information regarding size, location, number, and anatomic variants of pulmonary veins.
   - can be used to determine anatomic landmarks of right atrium.
     a. can be used to measure thickness of the crista terminalis and show the approximate location of the sino-atrial nodal artery.
     b. can be used to determine the boundaries of the Koch triangle and its adjacent structures.
     c. provides information on Eustachian valve and ridge.
     d. provides anatomic information of the cavo-tricuspid isthmus including size and anatomic variants, coronary sinus, and Eustachian ridge.
     e. provides information of the subthebesian pouch.

f. provides information of the inteatrial septum.

g. provides information of the septal components of the atrioventricular junction.

- provides information of the left atrium including the pulmonary vein orifices, the vestibule that surrounds the mitral orifice, and the appendage.

- can be utilized to monitor complications of radiofrequency ablation such as pulmonary vein stenosis.

2. MDCT can be useful prior to ablation of WPW syndrome.

3. Prior to cardiac resynchronization therapy, MDCT can be used to

- provide a comprehensive evaluation of the coronary venous anatomy.

- measure the orifice of coronary sinus and the target veins.

- evaluate anatomic barriers to the coronary sinus including the besian and Vieussens and valves, subthebesian pouch, coronary sinus diverticulum, unusual coronary sinus anatomy, vein of Marshall, and luminal narrowing of the crossing artery.

- determine the relationship between the neurovascular bundle and the target vein.

REFERENCES

1. Calkins H, Brugada J, Packer DL, et al. HRS/EHRA/ECAS Expert Consensus Statement on catheter and surgical ablation of atrial fibrillation. *Europace* 2007;9:335–379.

2. Haissaguerre M, Jais P, Shah DC, et al. Spontaneous initiation of atrial fibrillation by ectopic beats originating in the pulmonary veins. *N Engl J Med* 1998;339: 659–666.

3. Haissaguerre M, Jais P, Shah DC, et al. Electrophysiological end point for catheter ablation of atrial fibrillation initiated from multiple pulmonary venous foci. *Circulation* 2000;101:1409–1417.

4. Gage BF, van Walraven C, Pearce L, et al. Selecting patients with atrial fibrillation for anticoagulation: stroke risk stratification in patients taking aspirin. *Circulation* 2004;110(16):2287–2292.

5. Gage BF, Waterman AD, Shannon W, et al. Validation of clinical classification schemes for predicting stroke: results from the National Registry of Atrial Fibrillation. *JAMA* 2001;285(22):2864–2870.

6. Oral H, Knight BP, Tada H, et al. Pulmonary vein isolation for paroxysmal and persistent atrial fibrillation. *Circulation* 2002;105: 1077–1081.

7. Marrouche NF, Dresing T, Cole C, et al. Circular mapping and ablation of the pulmonary vein for treatment of atrial fibrillation: impact of different catheter technologies. *J Am Coll Cardiol* 2002;40:464–474.

8. Strickberger SA, Conti J, Daoud EG, et al. Patient selection for cardiac resynchronization therapy: from the Council on Clinical Cardiology Subcommittee on Electrocardiography and Arrhythmias and the Quality of Care and Outcomes Research Interdisciplinary Working Group, in Collaboration With the Heart Rhythm Society. *Circulation* 2005;111;2146–2150.

9. Daoud EG, Kalbfleisch SJ, Hummel JD, et al. Implantation techniques and chronic lead parameters of biventricular pacing dual-chamber defibrillators. *J Cardiovasc Electrophysiol* 2002 Oct;13:964–970.

10. Moss AJ, Hall WJ, Cannom DJ, et al. Improved survival with an implanted defibrillator in patients with coronary disease at high risk for ventricular arrhythmia. Multicenter Automatic Defibrillator Implantation Trial Investigators. *N Engl J Med* 1996;335:1933–1940.

11. The Antiarrhythmics Versus Implantable Defibrillators (AVID) Investigators. A comparison of antiarrhythmic drug therapy with implantable defibrillators in patients resuscitated from

cardiac arrest and near fatal ventricular arrhythmias. *N Engl J Med* 1997;337:1756–1783.

12. Bardy GH, Lee KL, Mark DB, et al. Amiodarone or an implantable cardioverter–defibrillator for congestive heart failure. *N Engl J Med* 2005;352:225–237.

13. Balaji S, Harris L. Atrial arrhythmias in congenital heart disease. *Cardiol Clin* 2002;20:459–468, vii.

CHAPTER 7

A Cardiac Surgeon's Perspective

Chittoor B. Sai-Sudhakar

C oronary artery disease is widely prevalent and is a major cause of morbidity and mortality in the Western world. The era of cardiac revascularization started in the 1950s with the introduction of the Vineberg procedure (direct implantation of the internal mammary artery into the myocardium) and has evolved into the current version of coronary artery bypass grafting (CABG), which is a frequently performed procedure worldwide. Traditionally, the vast majority of the revascularization procedures are performed by a median sternotomy utilizing cardiopulmonary bypass. However, with a greater understanding of the adverse systemic effects of cardiopulmonary bypass, and with the development of reliable cardiac stabilization equipment to facilitate accurate construction of the anastomosis, surgical revascularization is performed with increasing frequency as "beating heart surgery" or off-pump coronary artery bypass surgery (OPCAB). With a view to avoiding a median sternotomy, CABG is performed through a left anterolateral thoracotomy in the procedure of minimally invasive direct coronary artery bypass (MIDCAB) grafting. Developments in the field of port access and robotic technologies have led to totally endoscopic coronary artery bypass (TECAB) grafting, where the location and dissection of the coronary vessels are performed by visual feedback.

Annually, more than 800,000 patients undergo CABG around the world with more than half being performed in this country. While total arterial revascularization utilizing both internal mammary arteries and radial arteries is favored by many surgeons, saphenous vein grafts continue to be used by others. Among the arterial grafts, the left internal mammary artery graft to the left anterior descending artery has the best 10-year patency approaching 88% at 10 years.[1] This is especially true if the native vessel diameter is >2 mm with >50% diameter stenosis of the native left anterior descending artery. The saphenous vein grafts (SVGs) have patency rates of 60% at 10 years, with significant angiographic stenosis in 17% to 22% in the nonoccluded grafts at 10 years.[1] Early SVG occlusion occurs within hours or weeks after surgery because of technical inadequacies in 5% to 10% of grafts. Intimal hyperplasia and thrombosis account for the intermediate occlusion rate of 10% to 15% over the following year. After the first year, atherosclerosis results in vein graft degeneration. There is an SVG attrition rate of 1% to 2% per year between 1 and 6 years and 4% per year between 6 and 10 years after surgery.[2] With improved patient survival, there is a need for periodic surveillance of these grafts in addition to rapidly investigating any symptoms suggestive of coronary pathology (Fig. 7-1). Moreover, with ever-increasing rates of re-operative cardiac surgery, accurately visualizing the cardiac anatomy preoperatively is critical to devise the best operative strategy.

Coronary angiography remains the gold standard in defining coronary anatomy and graft patency. However, it is an invasive procedure and is associated with procedural risks including

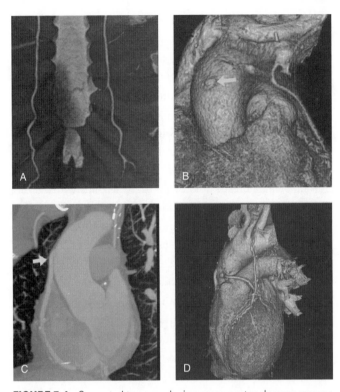

FIGURE 7-1. Computed tomography in coronary artery bypass surgery (CABG). **A:** Volume-rendered image of patent in situ bilateral internal thoracic arteries (ITA) prior to CABG. **B:** Volume-rendered image of occluded saphenous bypass grafts (SVG) and a left ITA graft. **C:** Curved multiplanar reconstruction showing patent SVG graft to right coronary artery (RCA). **D:** Volume-rendered image of patent left ITA graft from subclavian artery to left anterior descending (LAD). (See color insert.) (Reproduced from Topol EJ, Califf RM, et al. Textbook of Cardiovascular Medicine, 3rd Edition. Philadelphia: Lippincott Williams & Wilkins, 2006.)

stroke, native vessel dissection, acute myocardial infarction, ventricular arrhythmias, and puncture site morbidities such as hematomas and pseudoaneurysm formation. In addition, its deficiency in three-dimensional definition has led to the investigation of other noninvasive imaging techniques to define the overall coronary pathoanatomy. Initial attempts to utilize electron beam tomography and helical scan computed tomography were not encouraging because of motion artifacts, the need for prolonged breath holding, and image distortion due to metallic clips.[3,4]

Innovations in the field of computed tomographic imaging have led the development of multidetector computed tomography (MDCT) technology. MDCT allows for fast data acquisition in a single breath hold of 25 to 30 seconds with varying slice thickness, collimation, and Gantry rotation speeds following intravenous administration of 80 to 100 mL of nonionic contrast agent and a predetermined delay period to allow the contrast to reach the arterial circulation. Preprocedure β-blockade allows for a heart rate of <60 beats per minute since faster heart rates along with atrial fibrillation and ectopic beats impair the quality of images obtained. Image reconstruction and manipulation is facilitated by electrocardiographic-gated reconstruction algorithms.

EVALUATION OF THE NATIVE CORONARY ANATOMY

Martuscelli et al.[5] investigated the accuracy of MDCT in detection of significant (>50%) stenosis using a scanner equipped for 16 × 0.625 mm collimation and compared it with that of coronary angiography in 64 patients with suspected coronary artery disease.[5] Eighty-four percent of the angiographic segments were evaluable. Severe calcification, cardiac motion artifacts, poor opacification, and blending of the segments with veins hindered the evaluation of the remaining segments. In the segments which were evaluable, namely, vessels greater than 1.5 mm in diameter, multislice computed tomography (MSCT) had a sensitivity, specificity, positive predictive value, and negative predictive value of 89%, 98%, 90%, and 98%, respectively. MSCT had a 100% specificity and sensitivity in detecting total occlusion. Overall, MSCT detected 78% of stenoses detected by angiography. Cury et al.[6] demonstrated an excellent correlation between 16-slice MDCT and angiography in quantifying the degree of stenosis. However, MDCT tended to overestimate the stenosis. The evaluation of the coronary anatomy and the results were significantly better than those obtained with the 4-slice MDCT.[7] With the advent of 64-slice MDCT, Rubinshtein et al. analyzed its efficacy in the emergency room in evaluating patients with chest pain. They observed that emergency room MDCT had a high positive predictive value for diagnosis of acute coronary syndrome and a negative study predicted a low rate of major adverse cardiovascular event. In this study, only 4.6% of the coronary segments were of low image quality, testifying to improvements in MDCT technology and also aided by the low calcium burden.[8]

PLANNING FOR MINIMALLY INVASIVE BYPASS SURGERY

During the procedures of MIDCAB or TECAB, the visualization of the target vessels is limited and it is critical to identify the target vessel correctly and bypass it at the correct site. A common source of error is the bypassing of a large diagonal instead of the left anterior descending artery during minimally invasive surgery. In addition, the target vessels could be buried under epicardial fat, be covered by a myocardial bridge, run an intramural course, or be heavily calcified. Newer generation MDCT scanners have been shown to identify these variations in coronary anatomy better than coronary angiography.[9] These findings can dictate the type of surgery offered to the patients.

Coronary calcification is obscured by the dye used in angiography. In an open procedure, such areas can be palpated and anastomosis can be performed in the noncalcified segments of the coronary vessels. However, tactile feedback is absent in the minimally invasive procedures. Regions of coronary vessels burdened by calcification as evidenced by MDCT can be avoided for anastomosis.

EVALUATION OF GRAFT POTENCY

Re-operative cardiac surgery is associated with increased morbidity and mortality and the potential to inadvertently injure the bypass grafts. MDCT allows for the accurate three-dimensional visualization of the course of the left internal mammary artery graft in relation to the midline, location of other conduits (Fig. 7-2), and the degree of adherence of the right ventricle to the posterior table of the sternum. Unusual location of the grafts and their proximal anastomoses pose difficulties in evaluation by conventional angiography, especially in the absence of radioopaque markers for the proximal anasomoses. Faster data acquisition allows a manageable breath hold for the patient, allowing for visualization of the most proximal portions of the internal mammary artery grafts not seen in the early generation scanners. Martuscelli et al.[10] analyzed 285 conduits in 96 patients with 16-slice MDCT and compared the results to those obtained by conventional angiography. The sensitivity of MDCT in diagnosing significant stenosis was 96%.[10] Evaluation of graft patency and occlusion improved with the advent of 64-slice MDCT.[11] A recent analysis suggests that the sensitivity and specificity for graft occlusion approaches 100% across the studies, with only two cases of missed occlusions in bypass grafts, which were not visualized on MDCT. There are currently no reports of

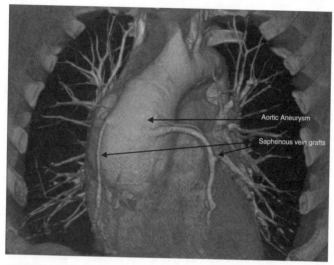

FIGURE 7-2. The 64-slice multidetector computed tomography demonstrates the patency of the grafts and the ascending aortic aneurysm.

false-positive occlusion. When diagnosing bypass graft stenosis, sensitivity ranged from 75% to 100%. Missed stenoses at distal anastomoses due partly to calcified wall plaque and membranous-like stenoses accounted for false-negative results. The specificity for diagnosis of stenosis of bypass grafts ranges from 89.3% to 100%. Poor opacification combined with small vessel size, vessel kinking, and surgical clip artifact account for false-positive results. The results from these eight studies of 1,169 coronary artery bypass grafts are similar to those obtained by coronary angiography. Several studies have reported that grafts not visualized on coronary angiography were visualized on MDCT, thus providing important additional clinical information.

However, assessment of native coronary arteries is impaired in the presence of atherosclerosis, calcification, and small diameter vessels. In addition, MDCT does not provide the flow characteristics of either the grafts or the distal run off. Arrhythmias, metallic clips on the side branches of the grafts, and higher heart rates continue to hinder adequate evaluation of the bypass grafts. Improved temporal and spatial resolution of the 64-slice CT scanner overcomes the artifacts caused by metal clips. Evaluation of in-stent stenosis by MDCT is difficult. Coronary stents are usually 2.5 to 4 mm in diameter. Blooming artifacts are produced by the metal in both the bare metal and drug-eluting stents. Cardiac motion compounds the problem. Partial volume effects lead to decreased visibility of the stent lumen, underestimate the luminal diameter, and overestimate the outer diameter. Inside the lumen of the stent, there is an increase in the attenuation, which can be minimized by utilizing submillimeter collimation and a sharp reconstruction kernel. With improving technologies areas, the larger diameter stents in the left main coronary artery and the proximal coronary vasculature can be analyzed for evidence of decreased luminal diameter due to intimal hyperplasia. The native coronary vasculature in the immediate vicinity of the stent is difficult to evaluate for stenosis because of beaming artifacts. In addition, beam hardening produces dark areas adjacent to the clips, stimulating stenosis especially at the anastomotic points.

With growing use of mechanical circulatory support devices in the management of heart failure, MDCT allows for the three-dimensional evaluation of the cannulas and reliably diagnose kinking of the outflow grafts.

MDCT is rapidly and effectively used as a one-stop test to evaluate the different causes of chest pain following CABG. Dual-source and 256-slice scanning allow for fast data acquisition, may further simplify the test, improve diagnostic accuracy, and eliminate the current limitations imposed by rapid hearts rates.

PRACTICAL POINTS

1. Cardiac CT, particularly 64-slice, has excellent diagnostic accuracy (sensitivity 100%) for occlusion and patency of arterial and venous bypass grafts.
2. The rate of nonassessable grafts is <5% with 64-slice MDCT.
3. Detection of anastomotic site and in the native coronary arteries is difficult after bypass surgery, in that overestimation of coronary obstruction occurs in the presence of coronary calcification.
4. The cost-effectiveness and safety profile of this technology means that it is a rapidly emerging tool in the assessment of coronary artery bypass grafts.

REFERENCES

1. Goldman S, Zadina K, Moritz T, et al. VA cooperative study group #207/297/364. Long-term patency of saphenous vein and left internal mammary artery grafts after coronary artery bypass surgery: results from a Department of Veterans Affairs Cooperative Study. *J Am Coll Cardiol* 2004;44:2149–2156.
2. Schwartz L, Kip KE, Frye RI, et al. Bypass Angioplasty Revascularization Investigation. Coronary bypass graft patency in patients with diabetes in the Bypass Angioplasty Revascularization Investigation (BARI). *Circulation* 2002;106:2652–2658.
3. Stanford W, Rooholamini M, Rumberger J, et al. Evaluation of coronary bypass graft patency by ultrafast computed tomography. *J Thorac Imaging* 1988;3(2):52–55.
4. Ueyama K, Ohashi H, Tsutsumi Y, et al. Evaluation of coronary artery bypass grafts using helical scan computed tomography. *Catheter Cardiovasc Interv* 1999;46:322–326.
5. Martuscelli E, Romagnoli A, D'Eliseo, et al. Accuracy of thin-slice computed tomography in the detection of coronary stenoses. *Eur Heart J* 2004;25:1043–1048.

6. Cury CC, Pomerantsev EV, Ferencik M, et al. Comparison of the degree of coronary stenoses by multidetector computed tomography versus by quantitative coronary angiography. *Am J Cardiol* 2005;96:784–787.

7. Kuettner A, Kopp A, Schroeder S, et al. Diagnostic accuracy of multidetector computed tomography coronary angiography in patients with angiographically proven coronary artery disease. *J Am Coll Cardiol* 2004;43:831–839.

8. Rubinshtein R, Halon DA, Gaspar T, et al. Usefulness of 64-slice cardiac computed tomographic angiography for diagnosing acute coronary syndromes and predicting clinical outcome in emergency department patients with chest pain of uncertain origin. *Circulation* 2007;115:1762–1768.

9. Herzog C, Dogan S, Diebold T, et al. Multi-detector row CT versus coronary angiography: preoperative evaluation before totally endoscopic coronary artery bypass grafting. *Radiology* 2003;229:200–208.

10. Martuscelli E, Romagnoli A, D'Eliseo A, et al. Evaluation of venous and arterial conduit patency by 16-slice spiral computed tomography. *Circulation* 2004;110:3234–3238.

11. Meyer TS, Martinoff S, Hadamitzky M, et al. Improved noninvasive assessment of coronary artery bypass grafts with 64-slice computed tomographic angiography in an unselected patient population. *J Am Coll Cardiol* 2007;49:946–950.

How to Set Up a Cardiac CT Lab

Laxmi S. Mehta

The success of a cardiac computed tomography (CTA) lab depends on lab design and workflow, marketing of services, and the financial equation. These factors all play a significant role and are interdependent and require attention in order to develop a successful lab. The upfront cost is high, which is complicated by low reimbursement rates, but with careful planning of the workflow and creative marketing, the procedure can be made cost-efficient and convenient.

SPACE ALLOCATION, EQUIPMENT, AND PERSONNEL

Much planning is required for space allocation. In-depth information regarding site planning and installation of equipment is provided by the computer tomography (CT) vendor, as each has its own specifications for room dimensions. The layout of the rooms may vary but typically include a lead-lined room for the scanner, a room for the operating console, and, if possible, a separate room for the generator and cooling systems. The floor, ceiling, and all the walls of the scanner room must be shielded with lead. These data provided by vendors detail the site planning for adequate function of the scanner, but these do not include the space required for preparing the patients prior to the test and monitoring after the scan. In addition, space is required for image archiving systems and workstations for image analysis and report generation, as well as for physician offices.

An efficient workflow is critical for a successful operation, as the number of patients scanned is higher and the patients are satisfied with a quick exam. Patient preparation is an essential component of the workflow, as the actual amount of time that the patient is on the scanner is minimal, but the time spent preparing the patient can be much longer as heart rate control is imperative for most scanners. Licensed staff (registered nurses) is required for obtaining intravenous access and administration and monitoring of prescan β-blockade therapy. Having at least two competent CT technologists also improves the workflow, while one technologist is processing the previous patient's images on a separate workstation, the other technologist is scanning the next patient. The CT technologists play a key role in the throughput of patients, quality of images, and daily maintenance of equipment. Image quality depends on two factors: (i) appropriate patient selection by the physician and preparation by the staff and (ii) implementation of suitable scan protocols with individual refinement of scan parameters by the technologist and the supervising physician. A physician program director should be assigned to manage the lab and the program, including protocol development and implementation and taking care of staff administrative responsibilities, to assess quality assurance of the lab, and to provide talks for physicians. He also needs to provide physician supervision onsite at all times to troubleshoot any scanning problems and to care for any medical emergencies that may arise, such as contrast allergies. A radiation safety monitor is needed to track the amount of radiation administered and help formulate plans to reduce amount of radiation exposure.

Efficiency of the lab is dependent on the effort and cohesiveness of the medical team.

Information technology support is paramount and requires broadband connections. After reconstruction of the images, the image data are provided in a standard digital imaging and communications in medicine (DICOM) format. Most CT scanner vendor packages include two-dimensional and three-dimensional workstations that operate on PC-based computers and frequently utilize a Windows operating system. These systems come with cardiac applications that vary from basic to advanced operating functions. Independent vendors manufacture workstations that are highly regarded with different functions and can be used instead of or alongside the workstations provided by the CT scanner vendor. Since many laboratories have more than one physician reading studies, much thought has to be put into whether to acquire more than one workstation. Another option is the availability of "thin-client" software that allows one to independently review images on a standard PC via intranet/internet connection to the main workstation.

In addition, thought has to be placed regarding data storage, as many states require archiving of images for at least 3 to 5 years after the scan. Since the amount of data acquired and needed for storage is enormous, standard media such as CDs or DVDs are insufficient and occupy much space. A more widely accepted method is PACS (picture archival and communications systems), which enables communication between systems and archival of images, including echocardiography and digital catheterization data.

MARKETING OF SERVICES

The service must be eloquently marketed to the medical community and to the general public. Close relationships need to be developed and maintained for a strong referral base. The referring practice will largely comprise of cardiologists but may also include primary care physicians, surgeons, and self-referred patients. Referring physicians need to be educated about the services available and the clinical utility, not only to boost the lab's volume but also to improve diagnostic usefulness. Marketing of services can be accomplished by physician-to-physician informal discussions, by informative lectures (continuing medical education or grand rounds), by open house of the facility, and by way of instructional printed resources. The marketing efforts should also focus on colleagues in the department as they are more apt to recommend a CTA if they were more knowledgeable about the technology.

After being scanned, a quick review of the images with the patient helps with the "wow" factor of the pretty pictures. Reviewing the coronary images with the patients also provides visual evidence for active intervention, such as lifestyle changes or the addition of medications. This guides the primary care physicians in pharmaceutical intervention and makes it easier to convince the reluctant patient to start certain medications (such as statins).

Another key aspect of marketing is report generation. The report should include the language used by cardiologists, as they are a large referring group, and color images of the salient findings. Some laboratories provide a CD with the report in order to demonstrate 3-D volume rendered images and angiograms of the coronary arteries to aid the referring physicians in making essential management decisions. To close the loop, feedback from the referring base is a critical step for enhancement of the day-to-day laboratory operations.

IMAGE INTERPRETATION

A "turf war" exists between cardiologists and radiologists regarding image interpretation. Cardiologists often feel that they have a better understanding of the cardiovascular system and can make more accurate assessment of the coronary anatomy, whereas radiologist are fighting a strong battle to prevent the loss of another imaging tool to cardiologists. This disagreement has caused an enormous division between these two specialties and in some centers has also involved vascular specialists who have a strong interest in vascular imaging. Each lab has to find its own solution to this conflict. Some centers have only radiologist interpreting the scan and others have only cardiologist interpreting the scan. The issue that remains for cardiologists is the liability of interpreting noncardiac pathology. Some cardiology groups have gone around the liability issue by collaborating with radiology groups. The typical agreement in this scenario is that the cardiologist reads the cardiac portion of the scan and the radiologist reads over the noncardiac structures. The split interpretation usually involves the cardiologist billing for the service and the radiologist receiving a fixed fee for his read, as of yet there is no ideal resolution for this disagreement.

FINANCIAL

Faced with Medicare cuts in reimbursement, every lab needs to assess whether to venture into investing in a CTA machine on its own, with other groups, or with hospitals. CTA clearly is a new technology with fancy pictures, yet it has to fit within the financial constraints of the investing group. The largest risk is early on as the initial investment for the equipment and staff is high with little turnover in patients. In order to stay financially sound, the scanner must be made available to scan noncoronary cases, such as peripheral vascular cases. Outlined in Table 8-1 are barriers that can impact the finances of a CTA lab.[1] One key factor is the rapid and ongoing evolution of CT technology, such as the type of scanners, number of detector rows, and

TABLE 8-1	Financial Realities Confronting Cardiovascular Computed Tomography

Equipment and space renovation is expensive

Historically there has been rapid depreciation in equipment value

Rapid technologic changes, often leaving prior generation scanners without purpose

Currently, limited referral population

Low volume of repeat imaging

Problems getting paid

Current CMS rates low relative to costs and work

Can negatively impact other imaging programs

CMS, Centers for Medicare & Medicaid Services.
Reprinted from Bateman T. Business aspects of cardiovascular computed tomography: tackling the challenges. *J Am Coll Cardiol Imaging* 2008;1:111–118, with permission from Elsevier.

availability of dual source scanning. As newer generations of scanners are rapidly available, the "old" equipment is swiftly depreciating with relatively inadequate function. Remodeling of office space, supplies, storage of data, service contracts all add to the expense of this technology. Another key expense is the salary and benefits of CT technologists, especially since the number of cardiac specialized technologists greatly lags the rapid growth of the technology. Table 8-2 shows the yearly expenses of an active CTA lab that utilizes a 64-slice CT scanner. Other things that complicate the finances are varying payment by insurers, need for large referral network, and infrequent repeat or sequential imaging of patients. The billing codes and reimbursement rates by insurance carriers are still a work in progress.

CTA is a rapidly evolving technology that provides the clinician with profound anatomical data. The clinical indications, "turf war," and reimbursement issues are dynamic and

TABLE 8-2	CT Expense Proforma

Assumptions

Staffing consists of CT technologist, nurse, clinical technologist, scheduler

Benefits/payroll taxes = 25% of salaries

Cost of CT scanner = $1.5 million, financed over the course of 5 y (lease with ownership end of lease)

Space rent of 800 sq ft @ $30/sq ft

Maintenance contract = $140,000/y for 2 to 5 y

Property taxes estimated @ $15,000/y in 2 to 5 y

Leasehold improvements @ $300,000 depreciated over the course of 10 y

Expense Proforma (5-y average)

Direct operating expenses

Salaries	$163,000
Benefits/payroll taxes	$40,750
Supplies/meds/contrast	$36,000
Office and administrative expense	$10,000
Professional fees	$5,000
Lease	$364,980
Rent	$24,000
Maintenance	$112,000
Insurance	$3,000
Marketing/advertising	$20,000
Property taxes	$12,000
Depreciation/amortization	$30,000
Total	$820,730

CT, computed tomography.

Reprinted from Bateman T. Business aspects of cardiovascular computed tomography: tackling the challenges. *J Am Coll Cardiol Imaging* 2008;1:111–118, with permission from Elsevier.

hopefully will resolve in the near future. The development of a robust CTA program is an exciting endeavor that requires insight not only in the technological features but also in business aspects of the program.

PRACTICAL POINTS

- Cost
  - The seven-figure cardiac CT scanner is not the only cost variable
  - The cardiac CT program should budget ≥$100,000 for each workstation
  - Information technology support including broadband connection
  - Data storage: DICOM storage, CT studies on optical disk or PACs
  - Personnel expenses
  - Space allocation including remodeling of existing office space
- Reimbursement and marketing
  - Reimbursement is decided at local level, third-party payments vary across the country
  - Marketing includes
    - Education of local physicians and requires educational talks to encourage physicians to reconsider their referral patterns
    - Prompt report generation to referring physician
    - Quick review of images including color reports to patients
  - Optimizing workflow
    - Short turnaround times including administration of IV β-blockers
    - Optimizing workflow in holding area
    - Radiation safety monitoring equipment
- Referrals
Are there enough cardiologists referring cases to generate volume of studies to support a break-even point?

- It is estimated that practices of >10 physicians are needed to sustain the investment.
- Estimates of minimum daily volumes vary from 4 to 8 scans to break even.
- "Auxiliary exams" may help defray costs, e.g., daily volume of two to three peripheral vascular studies, six to seven studies for calcium scoring (which takes seconds to perform and does not require β-blocker or coronary workstation).
- Noncardiac studies such as chest CT exams, head and neck CT studies, or general body CT, if the scanners have capability.

REFERENCE

1. Bateman T. Business aspects of cardiovascular computed tomography: tackling the challenges. *J Am Coll Cardiol Imaging* 2008;1:111–118.

Medicare Criteria for Cardiac Computed Tomographic Angiography

INDICATIONS AND LIMITATIONS OF COVERAGE AND/OR MEDICAL NECESSITY

Cardiac computed tomographic angiography (CCTA), also known as computed tomography of the heart and coronary arteries, or multidetector computed cardiac tomography, is considered reasonable and necessary for the evaluation of suspected symptomatic coronary artery disease (CAD) and for the detection of structural and morphologic intracardiac and extracardiac conditions.

Use of a CCTA is expected to avoid diagnostic cardiac catheterization. If high pretest probability of CAD exists, Medicare expects the patient to undergo invasive coronary angiography with appropriate percutaneous coronary intervention.

To establish CCTA's medical necessity, patient's case must meet at least one indication in the following two categories.

SYMPTOMATIC CORONARY ARTERY DISEASE

1. Evaluation of acute chest pain, unexplained dyspnea, or symptoms suggesting angina pectoris (such as jaw pain) when there is
   - intermediate pretest probability of CAD,[1] *and*
   - no electrocardiogram (EKG) changes to suggest acute myocardial injury or ischemia, *and*
   - normal initial cardiac markers.
2. Evaluation of chest pain syndrome when there is
   - intermediate pretest probability of CAD, *and*
   - uninterpretable EKG[2] or patient is unable to exercise, *or*
   - uninterpretable or equivocal stress test (exercise, perfusion, or stress echo).
3. Evaluation of intracardiac structures for suspected coronary anomalies.

SUSPECTED CARDIAC STRUCTURAL/ MORPHOLOGIC ANOMOLIES

1. Detection of intracardiac and extracardiac structures in
   - evaluation of cardiac mass (suspected tumor or thrombus) *or*
   - evaluation of pericardial conditions (mass, constrictive pericarditis, or complications of cardiac surgery), *or*

---

[1] Intermediate pretest probability of CAD by age, gender, and symptoms is between 10% and 90% as referenced in the ACCF/ACR 2006 Appropriateness Criteria for Cardiac Computed Tomography and Cardiac Magnetic Resonance Imaging.
[2] Uninterpretable EKG refers to EKGs with resting ST segment depression greater than or equal to 0.10 mV, complete left bundle branch block, pre-excitation, or paced rhythm.

- patients with technically limited images from echocardiogram, magnetic resonance imaging, *or* trans-esophageal echocardiogram.

2. Detection of morphologic intracardiac and extracardiac structures for

   - evaluation of pulmonary vein anatomy prior to invasive radiofrequency ablation for atrial fibrillation. While data are limited for three-dimensional reconstruction of the left atrium for ablations, there is broad consensus among cardiologists that these images, which are integrated and used in real time in the procedure room to shorten procedure time, improve therapeutic success and enhance patient safety, *or*

   - noninvasive coronary vein mapping prior to placement of biventricular pacemaker, *or*

   - noninvasive coronary arterial mapping, including internal mammary artery, prior to repeat cardiac surgical revascularization, *or*

   - detection of complex congenital heart disease, including anomalies of coronary circulation, great vessels, and cardiac chamber and valves, *or*

   - evaluation of coronary arteries in patients with new-onset heart failure to assess etiology.

LIMITATIONS

1. Coverage of CCTA is limited to computed tomography devices that process thin, high-resolution slices. Decreased resolution and slower rotation speeds result in a higher number of nonevaluable segments. At the current time, Medicare requires the multidetector scanner to have collimation of 0.625 mm or less, a rotational speed of 375 ms or less, *or* at least 64-slice detector design. Do

not submit studies from scanners that do not meet these requirements.

2. Medicare does *not* cover a screening CCTA for asymptomatic patients' risk stratification or quantitative evaluation of coronary calcium. Ultrafast CT scan of the heart (electron-beam tomography or electron-beam computed tomography) is *not* a covered service.

3. Simultaneous exclusion of obstructive CAD, pulmonary embolism, and aortic dissection ("triple rule-out") in the emergency department is *not* covered. In order to optimize imaging of the right coronary artery, contrast must be cleared from the right-sided chambers during acquisition, a process that leads to suboptimal contrast timing in the pulmonary arteries. Simultaneous rule-out of aortic pathology (at the low pitch needed to properly image the coronaries) mandates thicker slices in order to capture the total volume required in a reasonable breath hold. The increased slice thickness degrades coronary image quality.

4. For CCTA, patients must be able to lie still, follow breathing instructions, take nitroglycerine for coronary dilatation, and take a β-blocker or calcium blocker to achieve heart rates less than 70 beats per minute.

5. Prior to the initiation of a CCTA, there must be an imaging assessment of coronary calcification (calcium scoring). The physician must make an assessment of the anatomic location, degree and intensity of calcification, and impact of calcification on the utility of the test results. CCTAs performed on patients with elevated quantitative calcium scores that preclude accurate assessment of coronary anatomy are *not* covered by Medicare.

EXCLUSION CRITERIA

A. Contra-indications to contrast agent, including renal failure and dye allergy

B. Inability to lie flat

C. Pregnancy

D. Propensity to excessive artifact, including irregular heart rate (atrial fibrillation, frequent ectopics), tachycardia, inability to hold breath, pacing wires, and metallic valves

REPORTING CORONARY COMPUTED TOMOGRAPHIC ANGIOGRAPHY

Indication for examination

Imaging technique used
  Administration of contrast agents (type, dose, route)
  Vasodilator or β-blocker
  Workstation methods for image reconstruction
  Complications

Description of findings
  Overall description of image quality/diagnostic confidence
  Anomalies of coronary origin
  Right or left dominant system
  Location and size of any coronary artery aneurysm/dilatation
  Description of atherosclerotic narrowing for vessels ≥2 mm in
    diameter (CTA)
  Location of atherosclerotic narrowing by anatomic landmarks
  Diffuse or focal disease description
  15-Segment model may be used for description
  Noncardiac findings (e.g., adjacent lung fields, aorta)
  Ventricular size and function when requested if appropriate software
    is available

Limitations of the examination
  Heavy calcification (CTA)
  Motion abnormalities, arrhythmia
  Difficulties with contrast injection
  Summary statement/impression and recommendation

CTA, computed tomographic angiography.
From Bluemke DA, Achenback S, Budoff M, et al. Noninvasive coronary artery imaging: magnetic resonance angiography and multidetector computed tomography angiography: a scientific statement from the American Heart Association Committee on Cardiovascular Imaging and Intervention of the Council on Cardiovascular Radiology and Intervention, and the Councils on Clinical Cardiology and Cardiovascular Disease in the Young. *Circulation* 2008;118(5):586–606, with permission from Lippincott Williams & Wilkins.

EXPECTATIONS FROM A PHYSICIAN WITH LEVEL 2 OR LEVEL 3 TRAINING FOR CARDIAC CT

Know about

1. Various types of cardiac CT scanners available
2. Indications and risk factors that might increase the likelihood of adverse reactions to contrast media
3. Radiation exposure factors
4. CT scan collimation (slice thickness)
5. CT scan temporal resolution (scan time per slice)
6. Table speed (pitch)
7. Field of view
8. Window and level view settings
9. Algorithms used for reconstruction
10. Contrast media
11. Presence and cause of artifacts
12. Postprocessing techniques and image manipulation on work stations
13. Total radiation dose to the patient

CT, computed tomography.

From Budoff MJ, Achenbach S, Berman DS, et al., Task force 13: training in advanced cardiovascular imaging (computed tomography) endorsed by the American Society of Nuclear Cardiology, Society of Atherosclerosis Imaging and Prevention, Society for Cardiovascular Angiography and Interventions, and Society of Cardiovascular Computed Tomography. *J Am Coll Cardiol* 2008;51(3): 409–414, with permission from Elsevier.

TIPS TO MINIMIZE RADIATION EXPOSURE

Extensive coronary calcifications	• Quantity CAC score before CT angiography
	• Do not perform coronary CT angiography if CAC score is >800
	• Consider alternative diagnostic tests
Scan length	• Individually adjust the scan start and end of CT angiography, e.g., 1 cm cranially and caudally to the coronary arteries in the CAC scan
ECG-correlated tube current modulation	• Use in all patients with stable sinus rhythm
	• Consider more efficacious algorithms with a reduced tube current minimum, when available
100-kV tube voltage	• Use in all patients with a body weight of <85–90 kg (or BMI <30 kg/m^2)
	• Consider 100 kV also for timing bolus/bolus monitoring
Sequential scanning	• Consider in patients with a stable sinus rhythm and hear rate ≤63 beats/min

CAC, coronary calcium score; CT, computed tomography; ECG, electrocardiogram; BMI, body mass index.

From Hausleiter J, Meyer T. Tips to minimize radiation exposure. *J Cardiovasc Comput Tomogr* 2008;2:325–327, with permission. © Elsevier 2008.

LIFETIME ATTRIBUTABLE RISK OF CANCER INCIDENCE FROM A SINGLE COMPUTED TOMOGRAPHY CORONARY ANGIOGRAPHY SCAN*

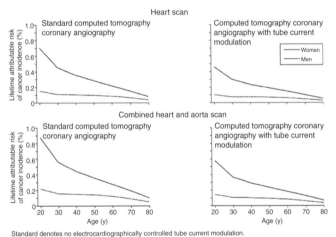

Standard denotes no electrocardiographically controlled tube current modulation.

The lifetime attributable risk (LAR) for a 20-year-old woman from a standard scan without electrocardiographically controlled tube current modulation was 0.70% (1 in 143). Risks were particularly high for women in their 20s and decreased markedly as a function of age. For a 40-year-old woman, the

*These estimates are based on the effective dose of 14 mSv in women and 9 mSv in men.

LAR was 0.35% (1 in 284); for a 60-year-old woman, the LAR was 0.22% (1 in 466); and for an 80-year-old woman, the LAR was 0.075% (1 in 1338). (From Einstein AJ, Henzlova MJ, Rajagopalan S. Estimating risk of cancer associated with radiation exposure from 64-slice computed tomography coronary angiography. *JAMA* 2007;298(3):317–323, with permission. © 2007 American Medical Association. All rights reserved.)

UTILITY OF MULTIDETECTOR COMPUTED TOMOGRAPHY PRIOR TO AFIB ABLATION

1. Anatomy of pulmonary veins including variants, ostial diameters of each vein, distance to the first-order branch, presence of accessory or supernumerary veins.

2. Dimensions of the left atrium and the presence of a thrombus in the left atrial appendage.

3. Anatomic course of the esophagus in relation of the pulmonary veins and posterior left atrial wall.

4. Presence of major anomalies including a common ostium to the superior and inferior veins, presence of persistent left superior vena cava, vein of Marshall, or anomalous pulmonary venous return.

Imaging Artifacts

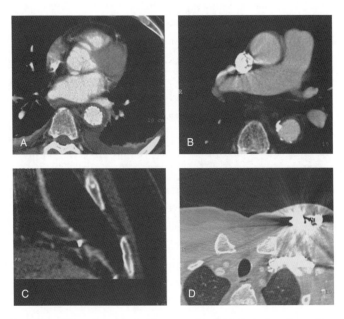

Imaging artifacts in computed tomography. **A:** A typical motion artifact at the ascending aorta in a nongated study. **B:** Contrast in the superior vena cava causing a radial streaking artificat. **C:** Surgical clips adjacent to a left internal thoracic artery bypass graft obscuring the anastomosis site to the left anterior descending artery. **D:** Pacemaker causing severe flash artifact.

CT imaging of the moving heart is based on a combination of multiple technical advances and stretches the temporal and spatial resolution of CT scanners to their limits. Imaging artifacts from any of these technical algorithms can render studies partially or completely uninterpretable or even produce false-positive findings. Recognition of these artifacts is thus vital to a clinical service. Motion or breathing artifacts will typically blur the contours of the heart, the coronary arteries, and the ascending aorta. Inconsistent triggering or arrhythmias may cause misalignment of adjacent slices. In combination with motion, partial scan reconstruction can cause streaks and low-density artifacts especially beside metal or calcium. Contrast in the superior vena cava can cause streaking artifacts. Edge-enhancing reconstruction filters can lead to artifacts along borders between very low and high density (e.g., the interface between lung and cardiac tissue) by smoothing out boundaries and assigning artificially high CT numbers to pixels along the edge zone. Finally, the "partial volume effect" is common in CT imaging: if an image pixel is only partially filled by a structure of very high attenuation (e.g. metal), the highest CT number will be assigned to the complete pixel, which will thus appear bright on the image. This will exaggerate the dimensions of high-intensity objects such as calcified plaque and cause significant difficulties in image analysis.

Image and text reproduced from Topol EJ, Califf RM, et al. Textbook of Cardiovascular Medicine, 3rd Edition. Philadelphia: Lippincott Williams & Wilkins, 2006.

MEDICARE REIMBURSEMENT

2009 Medicare Reimbursement for Cardiac Computed Tomography and Computed Tomographic Angiography Procedures (Reflects National Rates, Unadjusted for Locality)

CPT Code/ Application	Reimbursement Component	Hospital Outpatient Department[1]	IDTF or Physician Office[2,3]
CPT 0144T—non contrast cardiac CT Computed tomography, heart, without contrast material, including image post-processing and quantitative evaluation of coronary calcium	Technical	$105.01	Carrier priced/ CAP
	Professional	Carrier priced	Carrier priced
	Total	$105.01 + carrier priced	Carrier priced/ CAP
CPT 0145T— contrast cardiac CT/CT angiography Computed tomography, heart, with contrast material(s), including noncontrast images, if performed, cardiac gating and 3D image postprocessing; cardiac structure and morphology	Technical	$282.69	Carrier priced/ CAP
	Professional	Carrier priced	Carrier priced
	Total	$282.69 + carrier priced	Carrier priced/ CAP

(continued)

2009 Medicare Reimbursement for Cardiac Computed Tomography and Computed Tomographic Angiography Procedures (Reflects National Rates, Unadjusted for Locality) (Continued)

CPT Code/ Application	Reimbursement Component	Hospital Outpatient Department[1]	IDTF or Physician Office[2,3]
CPT 0146T— contrast cardiac CT/CT angiography Computed tomography, heart, with contrast material(s), including noncontrast images, if performed, cardiac gating and 3D image postprocessing; computed tomographic angiography of coronary arteries (including native and anomalous coronary arteries, coronary bypass grafts), without quantitative evaluation of coronary calcium	Technical	$282.69	Carrier priced/ CAP
	Professional	Carrier priced	Carrier priced
	Total	$282.69 + carrier priced	Carrier priced/ CAP

(continued)

CPT Code/ Application	Reimbursement Component	Hospital Outpatient Department[1]	IDTF or Physician Office[2,3]
CPT 0147T— contrast cardiac CT/CT angiography	Technical	$282.69	Carrier priced/ CAP
Computed tomography, heart, with contrast material(s), including noncontrast images, if performed, cardiac gating and 3D image postprocessing; computed tomo-graphic angiography of coronary arteries (including native and anomalous coronary arteries, coronary bypass grafts), with quantitative evalu-ation of coronary calcium	Professional	Carrier priced	Carrier priced
	Total	$282.69 + carrier priced	Carrier priced/ CAP

(continued)

CPT Code/ Application	Reimbursement Component	Hospital Outpatient Department[1]	IDTF or Physician Office[2,3]
CPT 0148T—contrast cardiac CT/CT angiography Computed tomography, heart, with contrast material(s), including noncontrast images, if performed, cardiac gating and 3D image postprocessing; cardiac structure and morphology and computed tomographic angiography of coronary arteries (including native and anomalous coronary arteries, coronary bypass grafts), without quantitative evaluation of coronary calcium	Technical	$282.69	Carrier priced/ CAP
	Professional	Carrier priced	Carrier priced
	Total	$282.69 + carrier priced	Carrier priced/ CAP

2009 Medicare Reimbursement for Cardiac Computed Tomography and Computed Tomographic Angiography Procedures (Reflects National Rates, Unadjusted for Locality) (*Continued*)

(continued)

CPT Code/ Application	Reimbursement Component	Hospital Outpatient Department[1]	IDTF or Physician Office[2,3]
CPT 0149T— contrast cardiac CT/CT angiography	Technical	$282.69	Carrier priced/ CAP
Computed tomography, heart, with contrast material(s), includ-	Professional	Carrier priced	Carrier priced
ing noncontrast images, if performed, cardiac gating and 3D image postprocessing; cardiac structure and morphology and computed tomo- graphic angiography of coronary arteries (including native and anomalous coronary arteries, coronary bypass grafts), with quantitative evalu- ation of coronary calcium	Total	$282.69 + carrier priced	Carrier priced/ CAP

(continued)

2009 Medicare Reimbursement for Cardiac Computed Tomography and Computed Tomographic Angiography Procedures (Reflects National Rates, Unadjusted for Locality) (*Continued*)

CPT Code/ Application	Reimbursement Component	Hospital Outpatient Department[1]	IDTF or Physician Office[2,3]
CPT 0150T— contrast cardiac CT/CT angiography Computed tomography, heart, with contrast material(s), including noncontrast images, if performed, cardiac gating and 3D image postprocessing; cardiac structure and morphology in congenital heart disease	Technical	$282.69	Carrier priced/ CAP
	Professional	Carrier priced	Carrier priced
	Total	$282.69 + carrier priced	Carrier priced/ CAP
CPT+0151T— add-on code Computed tomography, heart, with contrast material(s), including noncontrast images, if performed, cardiac gating and 3D image postprocessing; function evaluation (left and right ventricular function, ejection fraction and segmental wall motion) (List separately in addition to code for primary procedure)	Technical	$105.01	Carrier priced/ CAP
	Professional	Carrier priced	Carrier priced
	Total	$105.01 + carrier priced	Carrier priced/ CAP

CPT, current procedural terminology; IDTF, independent diagnostic testing facilities; CT, computed tomography; 3D, three-dimensional.

Courtesy of GE Healthcare, www.gehealthcare.com

Technical—is the facility payment; Professional—is the physician payment.

[1]Third party reimbursement amounts and coverage policies for specific procedures will vary by payer and by locality. The technical component is a payment amount assigned to an Ambulatory Payment Classification under the hospital outpatient prospective payment system, as published in Federal Register, Vol. 73, No. 223, November 18, 2008. The professional component is generally paid based on the Medicare physician fee schedule, but for Category III CPT codes, local Medicare contractors determine the payment rate. Amounts do not necessarily reflect any subsequent changes in payment since publication. To confirm reimbursement rates for specific codes, consult with your local Medicare contractor.

[2]Third party reimbursement amounts and coverage policies for specific procedures will vary by payer and by locality. The technical and professional components are generally paid based on the Medicare physician fee schedule, but for Category III CPT codes, local Medicare contractors determine the payment rate. To confirm reimbursement rates for specific codes, please consult with your local Medicare contractor.

[3]Per the Deficit Reduction Act of 2005, designated imaging services with a 2009 Medicare physician fee schedule technical payment (prior to geographic adjustment) that exceeds the comparable 2009 hospital outpatient prospective payment system (HOPPS) technical payment (prior to geographic adjustment), as published in Federal Register, Vol. 73, No. 224, November 19, 2008, will be capped at the 2009 HOPPS payment amount. For carrier-priced services subject to the DRA cap, the technical payment amount will be paid at the lower of the carrier-priced payment or the HOPPS payment rate. Accordingly, the global payment amount is the sum of the professional payment amount and the DRA capped technical payment amount.

Siemens Healthcare

SOMATOM DEFINITION™ DUAL SOURCE

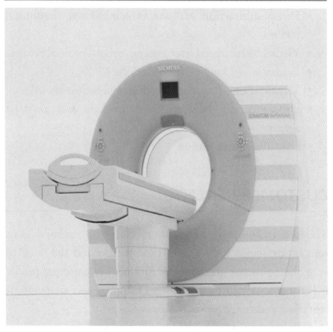

Courtesy of Siemens Healthcare.

PRODUCT DESCRIPTION

The Definition is the world's first dual-source computed tomography (CT) scanner, enabling CT acquisition with two x-ray sources and two detectors. Two spiral data sets acquired in a single scan provide diverse information, which enables clinicians to differentiate, characterize, isolate, and distinguish the imaged tissue and material.

CLINICAL ADVANTAGES

- Direct subtraction of bone in complicated anatomical regions
- Virtual unenhanced liver images without multiple scans
- Evaluation of lung perfusion defects
- Visualization of cartilage, tendon, and ligaments
- Differentiation between hard plaques and contrast agents
- Calculi characterization

CUSTOMER BENEFITS

The ideal customer for a Definition is one with a clinical focus on cardiovascular applications, dual energy, and the need to scan obese patients (dual power). Another key customer profile is Emergency Department, as the Definition sees tremendous workflow and triage power in this department.

- Faster than every beating heart
- Able to image all heart rates (including arrhythmias) without β-blockers
- Patient preparation, examination, and diagnosis in less than 10 minutes

- Full cardiac with half the dose
- Up to 50% lower dose at typical heart rates compared with today's most dose-efficient, single-source CT scanners
- One-stop diagnoses in acute care
- Easy, routine scanning regardless of size and condition of patients
- Emergency department triage of chest pain patients, making huge impact on operational cost and patient standard of care

WEBSITE

www.siemens.com/SOMATOMDefinition

Philips Healthcare

BRILLIANCE iCT

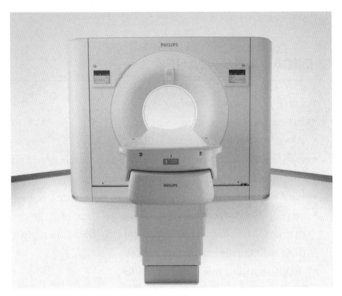

Courtesy of Philips Healthcare.

PRODUCT DESCRIPTION

Fast, noninvasive evaluation of chest pain patients in two heart-beats. iCT is so powerful that it can capture an image of the entire heart in just two beats while incorporating Philips technology that reduces radiation doses by up to 80%. The Brilliance iCT with 256 slices enables clinical excellence through the optimal combination of speed, power, coverage, and dose utility. It sets the benchmark for advanced cardiovascular imaging while simultaneously improving diagnostic accuracy and lowering the dose in all exams. Leveraging the power of essence technology, this configuration truly empowers new discoveries in clinical science.

CLINICAL ADVANTAGES

- Large area z-axis coverage—8 cm
- Fastest rotation speed in industry (270 ms)
- Power for any exam (up to 1,000 mA)
- ZFS tube technology improves z-axis resolution and eliminates many currently common artifacts
- Rate-responsive technologies adapt to the patient
- Step and shoot cardiac acquisition of data only at the desired phase, delivering approximately 80% lower dose than with conventional techniques
- Adaptive multicycle reconstruction

CUSTOMER BENEFITS

The Brilliance iCT system delivers the boost in performance and clinical capabilities that will not only expand clinical utility and enhance workflow but also improve image quality, diagnostic confidence, and patient experience for all cardiology and radiology imaging procedures.

- Consistent, accurate results for any exam, optimized for cardiovascular imaging
- Consistently accurate image quality for a more confident diagnosis
- Smart focal spot x-ray tube technology improves sampling density for enhanced spatial resolution in all exams
- Nano-Panel detector design enables fast and low dose examinations, which are particularly important for coronary artery imaging, lung scanning, and brain perfusion
- RapidView reconstruction provides high temporal resolution through adaptive, rate-responsive techniques to freeze patient motion

WEBSITE

http://www.medical.philips.com/us/products/ct/index.wpd

Toshiba America Medical Systems, Inc.

AQUILION ONE™

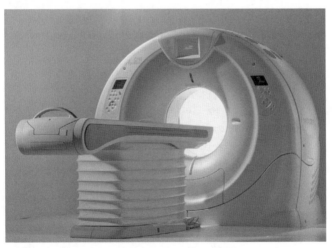

Courtesy of Toshiba America Medical Systems, Inc.

PRODUCT DESCRIPTION

The Aquilion family of premium computed tomography systems feature Toshiba's proprietary Quantum detector technology—the only detector which is able to acquire up to sixty-four 0.5 slices simultaneously. The Aquilion CFX series, available in 32- and 64-slice configurations, is specifically designed for cardio-vascular imaging, including the heart.

CLINICAL ADVANTAGES

- Essential images for noninvasive cardiac procedures and surgical planning
- For the first time, not only a three-dimensional depiction of an organ but also the organ's dynamic blood flow and function
- Coverage of up to 16 cm of anatomy using 320 ultrahigh resolution 0.5-mm detector elements
- Scan one organ—including heart, brain, and other organs—in one rotation at one moment in time
- No need to reconstruct slices of the organ captured from multiple points in time

CUSTOMER BENEFITS

With 4-, 8-, 16-, 32- and 64-slice customizable slice configurations, the Aquilion family delivers outstanding performance and clinical productivity to meet the needs of any size hospital or clinic. The Aquilion family shares a common platform with a clear upgrade path, making it the right decision today and ready for an easy upgrade tomorrow.

- Revolutionary patient care

- Reduced diagnosis time (from days and hours to mere minutes) for life-threatening diseases, such as stroke and heart disease
- Reduced exam time
- Reduced radiation and contrast dose
- Dramatically more accurate diagnoses

WEBSITE

http://www.medical.toshiba.com/Products/CT/DynamicVolume/

GE Healthcare

DISCOVERY CT750 HD

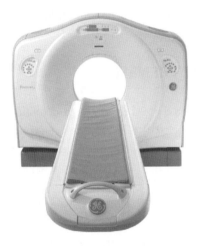

PRODUCT DESCRIPTION

The Discovery CT750 HD is the world's first high-definition CT with exceptional image quality for the heart and less dose, providing clinicians a technological and competitive edge in cardiac CT imaging. This system allows you to "see more" through unmatched image clarity and spatial resolution, "know more" via Gemstone Spectral Dual Energy imaging, and provide less dose for patients with all heart rates.

CLINICAL ADVANTAGES

- Exceptional vascular and cardiac image quality for detecting small lesions and small vessel assessment—renal arteries, coronary arteries, and peripheral vascular arteries
- Robust anatomical identification, segmentation, characterization, and quantification
- Up to 83% dose reduction for cardiac imaging

CUSTOMER BENEFITS

The Discovery CT750 HD is a high definition imaging CT scanner re-engineered to improve image quality enabling the visualization of greater anatomical detail and to provide the capability of reducing the radiation dose required for diagnostic studies.

- Improved spatial resolution, allowing the scanner to accurately quantify stenosis in coronary and vascular vessels
- Revolutionary advanced reconstruction algorithms that dramatically reduce dose by up to 50% as compared to predecessor CT systems
- Capable of advanced application techniques such as dynamic and spectral imaging offering the potential to enhance cardiovascular and vascular imaging by reducing blooming artifacts
- Image the coronary arteries or the entire heart in as little as 5 s that is repeatable across a wide range of heart rates

- SnapShot Pulse, prospectively gated scanning for less dose and improved image quality
- Complete ECG-gated study of the chest in a single breath-hold, in order to assist physician diagnosis of coronary artery disease, aortic dissection, and pulmonary embolism

WEBSITE

www.gehealthcare.com

INDEX